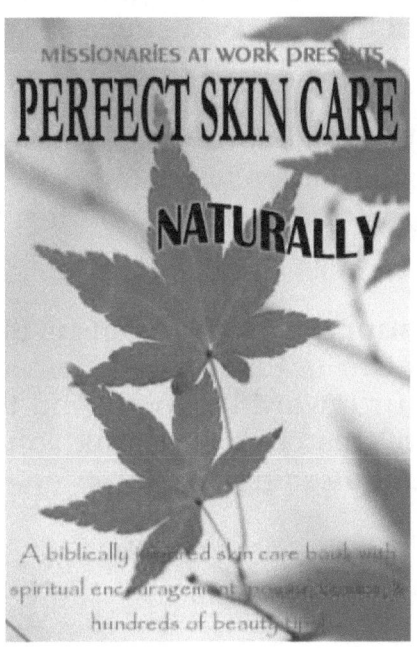

MISSIONARIES AT WORK PRESENTS

PERFECT SKIN CARE

NATURALLY

A biblically rooted skin care book with
spiritual encouragement, power scents, &
hundreds of beauty tips

Peace & Blessings

— ✳ —

Thank you to our Lord and Savior for continually allowing us to be a blessing to others that are much less fortunate. We thank GOD also for the wiliness of all the missionaries and volunteers who participated in this project. Thank you volunteers for giving of yourselves, for your very hard work, time and tears, and for so many skin care recipes and tips, you are wonderful and greatly appreciated, we pray the Lord will give us good success!

To some of M.A.W special friends, thanks to Werner Schuchner for the comic illustrations, Ray Torres for the web site Perfectskinnaturally.com and Weldon Brinson, Ruth Adegbola (Africa ministry) and Mari Van Wey Thank you for caring.

To all of M.A.W supporters, that join us in our mission to share the love of Christ throughout the world, thank you so much may your reward be great! And to everyone for the purchasing of this book we thank you and pray that it will be a continual blessing to all.

— ✳ —

THE SKIN

Your beautiful skin is the largest organ of your body. It measures approximately 20 square feet and weighs about 8 to 10 pounds. Your wonderful skin also requires one third of your body's circulatory blood for its healthy functioning. There are about 19 million cells per square inch of your beautiful skin. Now that's interesting, isn't it?

Your skin, as you know is a barrier against the world outside reflecting its own environment. Your skin environment includes what you are eating and what is going on inside of you as well as outside forces like stress and what products you are applying to your skin, and don't forget air pollution and other weather changes also affect your skin. Your wonderful skin is continuously working at removing waste or toxins from your body. The skin eliminating role is amazing. The body excretes one to two pounds of waste daily, through elimination and perspiring. When perspiration is inhibited, then the other body organs must work harder at eliminating impurities. The body then risks being placed in a toxic state that will show up on your beautiful skin.

While your skin is made of many layers, moisture retention and cell renewal occurs in the two upper layers, the dermis and the epidermis.

The dermis is where the major effects of the aging process take place. Its tissue consists of collagen protein and elastic fibers. Aiding and giving your skin its elastic quality.

The dermis contains thousands of tiny blood vessels. These little vessels carry nutrients and also help in removing waste from your system. The epidermis is the uppermost layer of the two. Containing no blood vessels, but small nerve endings and cells, these cells remain on your skin surface for a couple of weeks **and** are shed as new skin cells are made.

Your skin is constantly renewing itself but this process depends on the health and age of the person. As skin ages, the bonding that knits the skin cells closely together begins to break down. When this happens, dryness will occur followed by wrinkles and finally, sagging skin. To get or to keep a smooth dewy surface you must provide your skin cells with the right nutrients to help them stay healthy and happy. This begins inside you--for without proper nutrition hydration and rest, a dull appearance will result. To firm and tone exercise is recommended, there are some excellent exercises in this book that will help you tone and resist wrinkles and sags.

THE AGING SKIN

Under 22

With the onset of puberty, the hormonal balance in the body changes and during the teen years there is an increase production of sex hormones. These hormones will cause the sebaceous glands in the skin to enlarged producing an excess of oil on the skin. Because of the excess oil, pores may become clogged or blocked. When pores are clogged due to oil or bacteria an eruption may occur resulting in blemishes or acne. You'll find some wonderful hints in this book to help in this area.

TWENTY THREE TO THIRTY NINE

These are the reproductive years. Your pores look more refined but with time skin may begin to become slightly dry. Women who may have never needed a moisturizer before might now feel they need one. Most women may find there is less acne now except for an occasional flare up, but basically, skin should look strong and healthy.

Though skin should be in good condition, during these years women should avoid too much sun, cold, wind, and very hot water, all of which are drying to your skin. It is important to protect your skin from these natural forces. Also, around this time you might begin to notice little lines or tiny wrinkles. This is a good time to start a facial exercise program.

A WOMEN'S SKIN DURING Pregnancies

Though every woman's reaction to her pregnancy is different, there are some similarities. For instance, most women experience pigmentation changes in their body, on the face and the lips may appear darker. In addition, the breast nipples and the genital area may appear darker an enlarged. This is such a wonderful time, another benefit to being pregnant is the increase in blood circulation, which brings a radiance to your skin.

THIRTY NINE TO FIFTY

Your skin will need more of your attention now. If you've spent much time tanning in the past or simply an outdoors person spending more than usual time in the sun. You will now begin to see how too much sun may age you, and you will see the results of how you have treated your skin in the past, for it will now show.
You may start to see the first stages of wrinkles. To combat this you will need to start an exercise program right away, and stick to it to see results. And be sure to always wear moisturizer.

FIFTY AND OVER

During this time, your skin probably has gotten sensitive and perhaps a little dry. However, your skin can improve at any age, for it is always renewing itself. Be sure to continue your body and facial exercises to help tone and restore vitality to your skin. The pigmentation in dark skin offers a small amount of protection against the sun's UV rays. Dark skin also has other natural benefits. The natural collagen in dark skin which is arranged closely together, gives this skin more elasticity, thus, less wrinkles. Heredity or genes can make a difference in our skin. But there is wonderful hope we can all age beautifully. God has given us an abundance of knowledge to organically take care, restore and improve our skin. Rose Hip essential oil and rose the flower is excellent for mature skin renewal.

As you age, liver spots may begin to appear. They are caused by sun exposure. Your skin will show signs of aging, but take care of yourself and your skin will look good right up to a ripe old age. You are never too old to take care of or repair your beautiful skin.

One's ethnic heredity has a lot to do with the amount of damage the sun may do in a person's lifetime. For example, people from a European or Scandinavian line are the most susceptible to sun damage. People from a Mediterranean background are a little less susceptible, while Latin and Asian people have a skin somewhat similar to dark or African skin. However, do enjoy the sun! From it we receive nourishing nutrients, especially vitamin D, which helps to fight cancer forming agents.

For thou hast possessed my reins; thou hast covered me in my mother's womb. I will praise thee; for I am fearfully and wonderfully made;

Psalm 139

On top of the Rainbow

Looking over the rainbow where eagles fly
Running my race with my eyes on the sky
Pressing forth though cares and distractions
Surround me

I cast them on his shoulders and I run free
Climbing the rainbow where going in
Like Jonathan armor bearer, I go with him
The work is hard his yolk is easy

Walking in the vision that stayed before me
On top of the rainbow just me and my LORD
My lamp is lit it's full of oil

My dreams and battles he helps me to win
On top of the rainbow with Jesus
My true friend

YOUR SKIN TYPE

One of the first steps to taking care of your skin is to know you skin type, and not to use harmful products on it. The main categories for skin types are normal skin, dry skin or oily skin. Most skin is a combination of the three. Heredity plays a big part in your skin type, as you know, but your health habits and environment contribute to your skin's overall health as well. For example, people living in very warm dry states may commonly have dry skin because of the frequent sun exposure. Living in very cold weather will also give you dry and somewhat rough skin if you don't take care of it. Other places where it rains more frequently, skin is supple because of the moisture in the air and less sun exposure.

NORMAL SKIN

This skin type is found mainly in the young or older individuals attentive to their health and their skin. Normal skin type shows a good balance of oil and moisture retention, including a general sign of good physical health. Normal skin also displays small to medium sized pores and a smooth appearance.

Easy quick wash, in the palm of your hand
Mix 1/4 teaspoon of your favorite clay or oatmeal mask and 1/4 teaspoon tea tree oil or vitamin E oil, apply to dampen face, work up lather and rinse clean.

OILY SKIN

Oily skin is often a hereditary trait. This skin type normally has large pores and most commonly an overall shiny appearance. Oily skin is prone to clogged pores and blocked hair follicles creating acne and blackheads. Herbs like Golden Seal and Echinacea is excellent for this skin type. These herbs will help bring a natural balance to the skin.

Easy quick wash, in the palm of your hand
Mix 1/4 teaspoon your favorite over the counter clay or oatmeal mask and1/4 teaspoon lime juice or tea tree oil, apply to dampen face work up a lather and rinse clean.

DRY SKIN

Dry skin is often sensitive with poor elasticity. It doesn't normally break out in pimples or get blackheads. It exhibits a dull flaky appearance. This flakiness is sign of dehydration, which may increase the tendency towards fine lines and wrinkles because of the lack of moisture in the skin. Pores are normally small with this skin type and is negatively affected by hot water and very cold weather.

Easy quick wash, in the palm of your hand,
Mix 1/4 teaspoon your favorite over the counter clay or oatmeal masque and 1/4 teaspoon vitamin E oil or grape seed oil, or try your favorite essential oil apply to dampen face, massage, work up a lather and rinse clean, apply moisturizer.

COMBINATION SKIN

Combination skin is the most common skin type and includes both dry and oily qualities.
You can recognize combination skin normally by an oily T-zone (forehead, nose, cheeks and sometimes chin) while the jaws may be slightly dry. It is really two different types of skin, and should be cared for accordingly. The goal is to moisturize the dry areas and to stabilize the oily areas. Vitamin A is excellent for helping to balance and hydrate the skin.

SENSITIVE SKIN

Sensitive skin is delicate and dry. It is easily irritated and should be treated very mildly, with non-soap products. This skin type will react negatively to synthetic chemicals in your care products. Exposure to the sun, cold and windy weather may be damaging to this skin, causing it to age too quickly. Chamomile oil, cucumber seed oil, and orange blossom oil can be very helpful to this skin type.

ECZEMA SKIN

Eczema skin is a dry skin condition in which there is itching of the skin wherefore a rash may develop due to irritation to the dry skin. There may be blistering and oozing. Try to keep this skin type very moistened, to avoid outbreaks.
A cleanse or fast to clean and flush your system is advised. Rose flower is excellent for mature or dry skin.

ROSACEA SKIN

Rosacea is a skin disease that normally appears on the Face, forehead nose cheeks and chin, (T zone)causing redness and swelling. The skin may also have visible blood vessels. Comfrey or chamomile Steam baths are recommended and organic vitamin C skin products.

PSORIASIS SKIN

Psoriasis is a disease of the immune system that reflects on the skin with itchy scaly rash-like patches. Tree oil and chamomile steam baths would be an indulgent this skin would appreciate.

Both Rosacea and Psoriasis skin can flare up when provoke or triggered. Therefore, the thing is to figure out what triggers your flare ups and to avoid that annoyance or make peace with it if at all possible. Flare ups may be related to stress; it is important to avoid irritating or scrubbing the skin with exfoliates. Instead, use fragrance-free cleansers, luke to cool water rather than hot water on skin, as hot water can be irritating and will not help the symptoms.

A cleanse or fast is recommended with lots of water to flush and clean your system. Natural organic moisturizers that will help include Grape Seed oil, Flag seed oil (contains omega 3) which is highly recommended to relieve symptoms, peanut oil, mango butter, papaya seed oil. In addition the Fever few (flowers) plant in the chrysanthemum family are quite helpful in calming symptoms. Include some of these natural oils and ingredients in your homemade products.

You will find the ingredients for making your natural skin care products at your local grocery or health food store.

A few anti-aging antioxidants

Here a few anti-aging antioxidants to help us better care for our skin. They are found in our foods ,and you can create your skin care products using the ingredients that come from your kitchen; we can create cleansers, lotions and creams that are full of antioxidants that will help our skin cells to stay healthy, so that they may easily renew themselves. Your skin will drink up every drop of nourishment and you will be left with fresh vibrant skin.

Alpha Tocopherol is most own as vitamin E, it helps in skin cell renewal. Studies also show it to be good for the heart, wheat germ, olives, nuts, pumpkin, and sunflower seeds are an excellent sources of vitamin E.

Vitamin C also known as ascorbic acid, increases collagen production, Include vitamin C in your diet and there will be fewer wrinkles. Vitamin C is found in citrus fruits, tomatoes etc.

Vitamin A beta carotene is an anti aging antioxidant that will aid your skin in skin renewal and will help retain your natural moisture. An excellent reason to eat your vegetables!

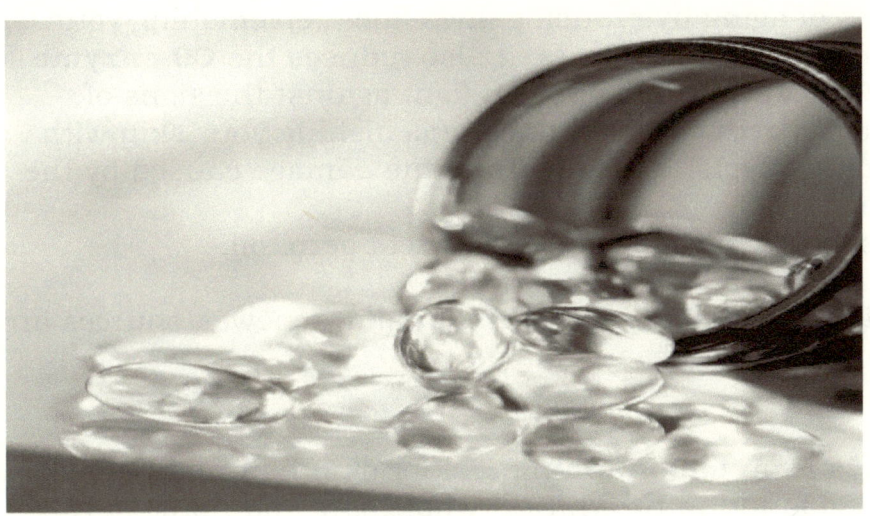

Vitamin B will help your skin to stay clear and smooth it is very important for skin renewal. You will find vitamin B in milk, eggs yolks and brewer's yeast.

Vitamin E oil, has an healing effect to the skin, it helps reduce and soothes wrinkles, moistens and tones skin. Wheat germ oil, avocado and egg yolks contain this vitamin.

COenzyme Q10 vitamin oil, helps you fight against the signs of aging by reducing fines lines replenishing your skin with firming effects. It also reduces the **CO enzyme Q10 vitamin oil,** helps you fight against the signs of aging by reduces fines lines replenishing your skin with firming effects. It also reduces the damage caused by the sun.
It is found in egg whites and wheat germ oil.

Silicon, a mineral necessary for skin renewal, sources are whole oats and beer.

Silica is an important mineral for skin hair and nails. It is also found in brown rice, whole oats and horse tail extracts.

Silica or Silicon, the health of your skin depends on It. This mineral is essential to your all around good health. Traces of this mineral are found in every organ and cell of the human body with the greatest amount being found in the skin and hair. So needless to say, Silica (silicon) is essential for strong bones, strong hair & nails, and youthful healthy skin. Foods with Silica are Wheat bran leafy green vegetables, beets soybeans, and pork rinds etc.

Zinc will promote your natural collagen that gives your skin its elasticity. Sources: fresh fruit and vegetables.

What's in your moisturizer?

Is your moisturizer good enough for your precious skin?
You are the judge.
Moisturizing lotions and creams are light emulsions of
water and oil that are supposed to protect your skin from
harsh elements and aid in giving moisture to your skin.
They contain 50-90 percent water. Here is list of some
common ingredients used in most moisturizers.

SODIUM LAUREL SULFATE

This ingredient found in many beauty products. However,
it is linked to hair loss and allergic reactions.

MINERAL OIL OR PETROLEUM PRODUCTS

These products appear to be moisturizing when applied
but they clog your pores and deprive your precious skin
cells of oxygen needed for new cell growth.

LANOLIN

This product is used to protect the skin, but people with
sensitive skin may develop a rash, lanolin comes from
sheep wool, so there is a slight possibility it could carry
pesticides on to your skin.

PROPYLENE GLYCOL
This ingredient is very popular; however, it may give
sensitive skin allergic reaction.

There is a rule we go by that is if you can't eat it or
pronounce it, it shouldn't be on my skin, going into my
system.

KAOLIN AND BETONITE
Depletes your skin of moisture and oxygen,

STEARIC ACID a colorless, odorless wax like fatty acid
found in animal and vegetable fats.

GENTLE MOISTURIZERING

Here are some natural moisturizers that are kinder to your skin, try any of these in your toner, lotion or creams.

EXTRA VIRGIN OLIVE OIL, softens & replenishes skin will look dewy to touch.

GRAPE SEED OIL, softens skin, great for normal to oily type.

WHEAT GERM OIL is an excellent moisturizer offering antioxidant benefits especially good for sun damaged skin.

PANTHENOL, a pro-vitamin B derivative that retains water, reduces wrinkles, is good for hair, and nails.

VITAMIN A and Vitamin E oil improves the texture of skin and stimulates new skin cell growth and offering antioxidant benefits helping your skin to fight against signs of aging.

ALMOND OIL will smooth and soften your beautiful skin.

ALOE VERA aids in retaining water and encourages cell repair and new growth. Helps in nourishing, tone, and soothes.

APRICOT OIL is excellent soothing oil for delicate dry skin.

AVOCADO OIL rich in protein A, D and E nutrients. Good for normal to dry skin, helps moistens and reduce wrinkles.

BLACK CURRANT SEED OIL
Has healing benefits for dry skin. And will help restore the health of damage skin cells.

CANOLA OILS A light oil that easily absorb through the skin Great massaging oil.

CASTOR OIL a thick oil from ancient days pressed from the castor bean. This oil is a natural emollient to the skin as it penetrates it makes skin soft.

CHAMOMILE OIL improves the texture and elasticity of the skin, also helps to calm very dry skin.

COCO BUTTER or COCOA OIL
Provides a natural fatty acid that moistens and soften your skin.

COCONUT OIL easily absorbs by the skin, will moisten and soften skin

COLLAGEN GEL adding collagen to your skin helps in nourishing it and improves the health of skin cells.

Cucumber seed oil is excellent for mature delicate dry skin.

CYPRESS OIL, good for oily skin and reduces signs of cellulite and helps in relieving varicose veins, essential oil

EMU OIL helps fade scars and has wonderful moisturizing benefits. Great massaging oil aids in easing muscle aches & pains.

FRANKINCENSE and MYRRH OIL (essential oils) are very effective in reducing fine lines and wrinkles when combine together.

GERANIUM OIL an essential oil good for oily skin

GLYCERIN helps in maintaining moisture and aids in softness.

JASMINE OIL an essential oil can be use as a softener. Be sure to dilute.

JOJOBA OIL is great moisturizing oil with an excellent shelf life. The skin is soften and renewed as it quickly absorbs this moisturizer.

LAVENDER OIL has healing benefits for all skin types, tones skin, and an essential oil.

LEMON OIL just a little is good for oily skin an essential oil.

NEROLI OIL and ORANGE BLOSSOM OIL helps in regenerating skin cells good for dry or sensitive skin. Helps you balance your skin and it encourages skin cell renewal an essential oil

PATCHOULI OIL, makes a great toner or astringent, has additional cleansing benefits good for blemishes.

PRIMROSE OIL, just a little is needed excellent moisturizer, good for normal to dry skin.

ROSE HIP OIL replenishes your skin and reduces fine lines. Essential oil

ROSEMARY OIL will help to stimulate your skin cells into rejuvenating themselves. Excellent for dry skin, essential oil

ROSE OIL is very soothing and can be like medicine to dry or sensitive skin also helps reduce large capillaries, essential oil

SANDALWOOD OIL will help your skin retain its moisture, an essential oily

SESAME OIL is very soothing and is easily blended with other oil. Moistens and helps even skin tone

SHEA BUTTER is a great moisturizer that can be blended with other oils in order to increase the benefits.

SUNFLOWER SEED OIL light oil rich in vitamin A and E,

ESSENTIAL TEA TREE OIL
Is a gentle antibiotic essential oil, great for oily skin and for acne skin flare ups?

WHEAT GERM OIL, an excellent moisturizer offering antioxidant benefits. It is especially good for sun damaged skin.
For normal to dry skin, apply your moisturizer to damp skin. Your skin will absorb your moisturizer quickly and will stay moisten longer.

For oily skin, apply your toner oil or lotion to dry skin.

Carefully use essential oils they should always be use sparely for they are highly concentrated and may irritate. Be sure to dilute and to test an area first before applying. Concentrated oils should be kept away from children, and of course, any open wounds including your eyes.

Natural moisturizers are found at your local health food store. Have fun and experiment by mixing two or three or more natural oils together to create the perfect moisturizer for yourself add fragrance according to your preference have fun and be creative it is very satisfying to be able to make your own skin care products that work for you.

NOTE: be sure to test an area first to see if you are compatible with the oils you have chosen. By taking a small diluted amount and apply to skin, not on the face, then wait to see if there is a negative reaction

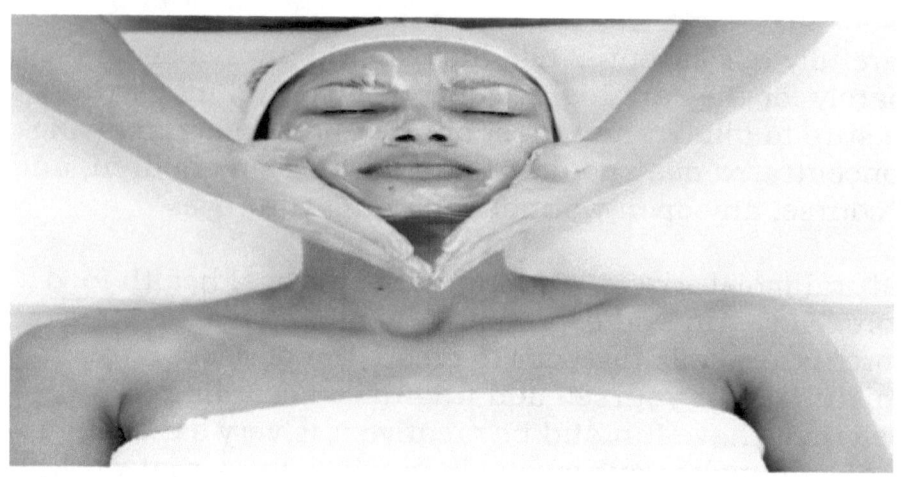

Jesus a knight and shining armour
and the answer to a girl dreams

CARING FOR SKIN WITH ACNE

Cleansing three to four times a day should keep the face clear of debris. After cleaning, follow with a toner, preferably mineral water and lemon or lime juice. You can use a medicated ointment if need be that consist of Benzoyl-peroxide. Heavy lotions or moisturizing creams are a no no, of course. Try never to squeeze or pop a pimple as this may cause an infection and possible scaring. Be attentive to keep lotions that clog your pores away from your skin. Wearing your hair back off your face would help and also avoid touching your face with your fingers throughout the day.

Frequent facial scrubs or exfoliate may cause inflammation and stimulate your oils glands. Moreover, you may feel that a tan helps your skin look better. But in fact a tan will not help your acne. Excess sun exposure will thicken your skin and may cause your pores to clog more frequently, thus making your acne worse. Simply try to detoxify the skin often Lifting bacteria and excess oil from your pores is needed to gain healthy skin. An apple cider vinegar or lime astringent is recommended for this, also steam facials, seaweed and clay masks.

1) *Sallys skin woke her with a song this morning.*

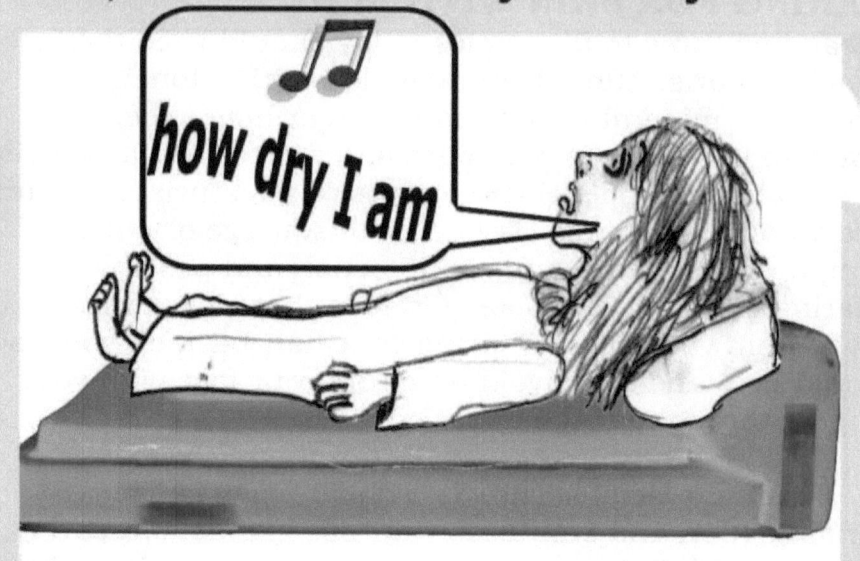

2) *dont let this happen to you*

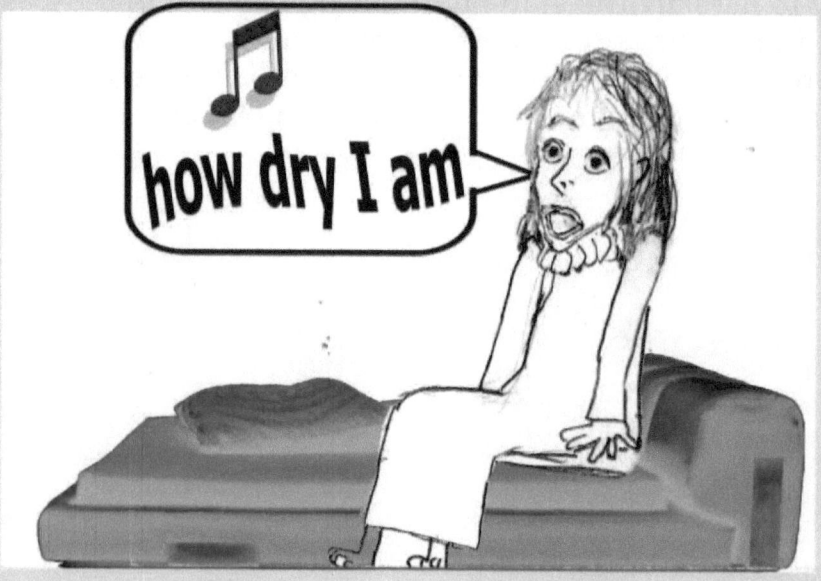

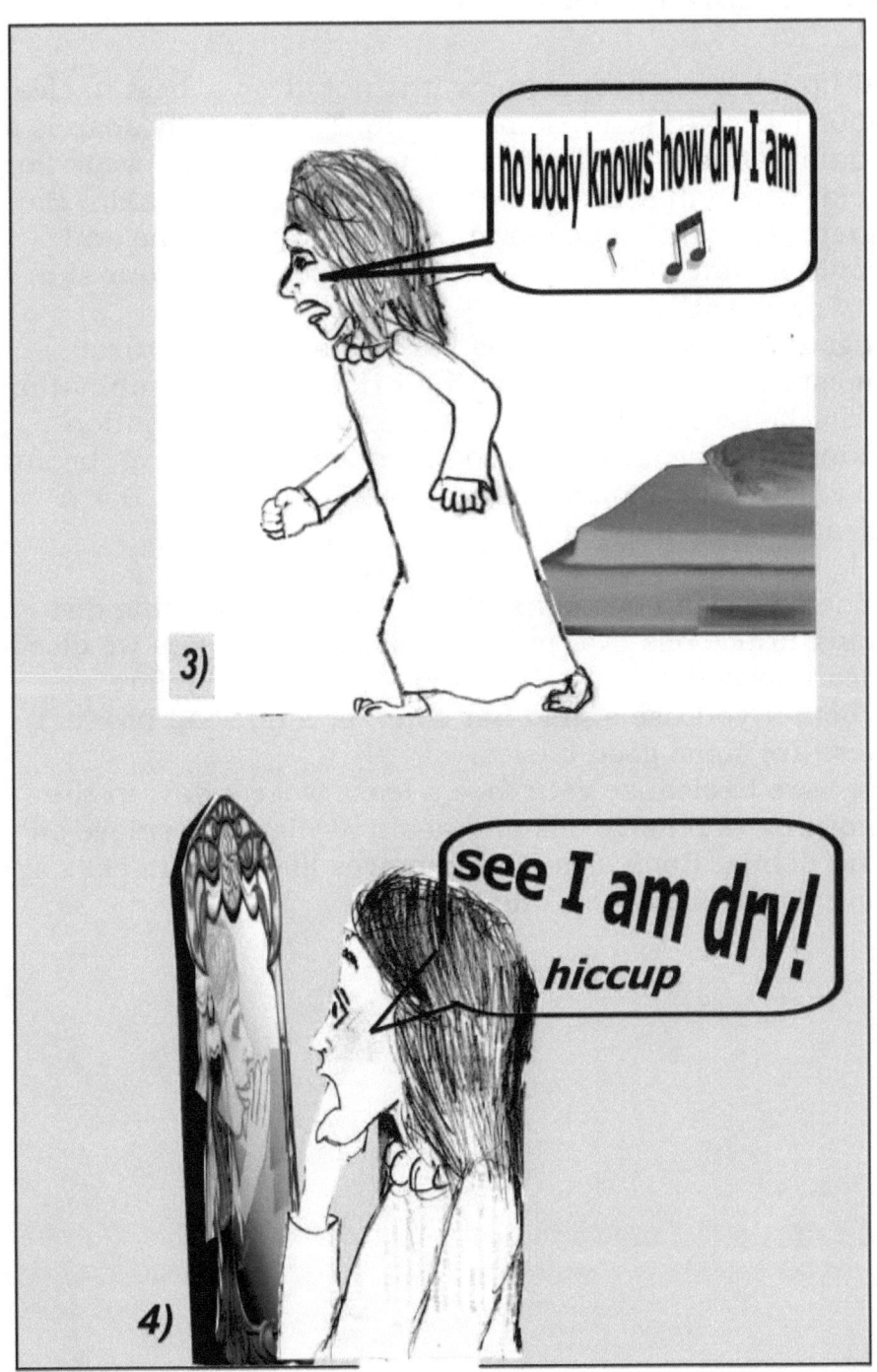

CLEANSING THE FACE

Although most people know it is not always, best to clean your face with soap, some still do. Traditionally soap is a combination of a strong alkaline product and a weak fatty acid, which may be too harsh for your delicate skin. Bar soaps, containing deodorants are highly alkaline and could irritate your precious skin, especially if your skin is dry or sensitive.
A good non-soap cleansing bar containing a natural moisturizer is recommended for normal and combination skin, being sure to moisten dry areas in combination skin. A bar cleanser is recommended for oily skin, be sure to follow with a toner (astringent). For dry skin, use a cleansing cream or milk.

When we clean our skin we are not only removing dirt and surface oils that may be clogging our pores we also clean away dead and damaged skin cell. Therefore, whether you use a mild bar soap, or a no soap product, here are some good basics.
Be sure to cleanse your face a least twice a day, in the morning to remove oils and again at night to remove oil and debris. Each cleansing removes lifeless skin cells and reveals the fresh new ones.

When cleaning the face, moisten it first with a few splashes of water or with a soft damp cloth. Then using your fingertips, apply cleanser gently in upward circular movements, lifting any surface debris and stimulate skin renewal. Rinse with warm water, following with cool splashes to help close your pores.

Never go to sleep with make up on, as you know, you are clogging your pores, and depriving them of oxygen by doing so. The results may be a pimple outburst and eventually a dull rough skin surface, also never apply make up to unclean skin.

Be sure to remove make up before any strenuous exercise, as you don't need anything obstructing your breathing neither does your skin
When deciding on a cleanser look for fragrance-free products. Fragrances may irritate skin.

When cleaning your face be careful not to pull your skin, as little pulls here and there may stretch your skin, so be gentle, and after bathing when possible let your skin air dry, or pat dry.

Note: the following all natural skin care recipes were developed to promote and restore healthy skin, with continuous use.
Now before you beginning thoroughly clean and sanitize your work area and utensils.

BECAUSE

Because I love him I bless the poor
Because I love him I thirst for more
More of him that makes me salty
Then others thirst for him like me

Because he loves me my cares are gone
He holds them now I sing a song
I'm so grateful he's loving me
I just believe and I was set free

The Love of GOD is shed abroad
Because he loves us one and all
And it's the love of God in me
That makes me care for those in need

The Love of GOD is loving you
The savior's love is always true
And no one knows you exactly
As the maker of you, you see

Because he loves you the sun will shine
Because he holds your future and mines
And life is given more abundantly
Oh the Love of GOD for you and me

EASY CARE NATURAL CLEANSERS

Tea cleanser

1 cup diluted brewed chamomile
2 tablespoon vegetable glycerin
A couple drops of essential tree oil
Two drops lemon oil
Lemon peels
Place ingredients in glass container shake before each use.
For oily skin, this cleanser will help fight against acne, and calm skin.

This is one of our favorite cleansers it is gentle, easy to make. Refrigerate it and it will keep a couple of weeks.

123 facial Cleanser

One tablespoon ground powder oats
Two drops of Geranium essential oil
Three tablespoons milk, (cow, coconut or soy)

Whip ingredients until creamy with a hand mixer.
 Then apply to face in gentle upward circular motions..

For normal to oily skin

In Haiti, we were in the hot sun most days. This cleanser
saved my skin I believe. I have depended on this wash
repeatedly to clean and balance and nourish my skin in
one-step. It's not drying and I love that! I let the oats soak
in the milk a little then add oil, and if I have time I will
warm it slightly this is my indulgence.

Milk treat

One tablespoon ground powder oats
Three tablespoons coconut milk
½ tablespoon avocado oil
Two drops of gardenia oil

Apply gently to face

For normal and dry skin

This wash certainly is a treat while you are cleaning your beautiful skin your cleanser is restoring natural oils and luster to your skin.

Basic wash

One Cup carbonated mineral water
One tablespoon vegetable glycerin
One tablespoon aloe vera
½ tablespoon corn meal
One teaspoon extra virgin olive oil
Two or three drops of rose hip oil
Two drops of rose oil

─ ✳ ～

Mix all ingredients together shake well before each use. Normal to dry skin will love this cleanser.

I told my grandmother from Holland, I wish I had her skin it is always so soft and fresh looking and she looks so much younger then she is. Then she told me her secret, it's this wash I substitute here and there depending on what's available, but this is the basic wash. I bought this recipe to my small group, we all love it, and the proof is in our glowing faces.

The wise woman builds her house
but with her own hands
The foolish tears hers down

Proverb 14

─ ✳ ～

Berry delight

Puree 3 or 4 strawberries
One ½ tablespoon cooked oats
One teaspoon honey
¼ teaspoon fresh chopped ginger
Buttermilk

Mix all ingredient together except buttermilk with hand mixer till creamy, apply to face in gently upward strokes, rinse with buttermilk, for all **skin types,** cleans and tones the skin.

This is a lovely cleanser, it hydrates my skin.
I make up enough to last a few days, and it is very refreshing.
Refrigerate, or warm slightly before use, it really is a delight to use after returning from the fields, my skin drinks in all the nutrients immediately, this wash cleans and restores my skin to a healthy glow.

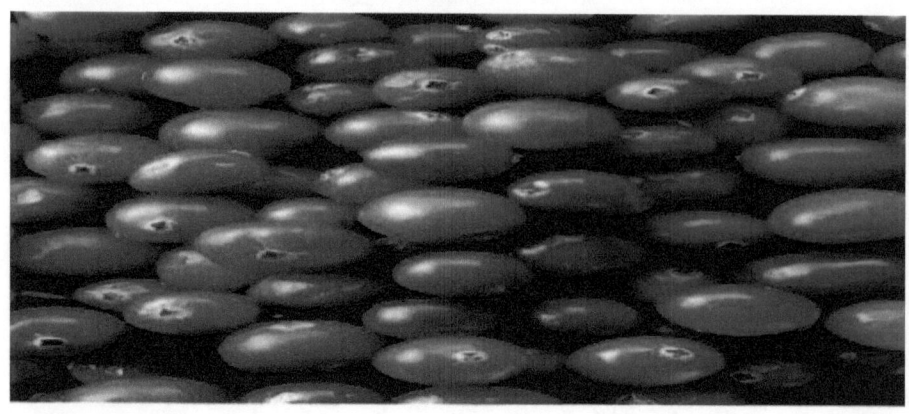

Berry delight #2

Puree 3 or 4 strawberries
One tablespoon plain yogurt
½ teaspoon tea tree essential oil
A drop of rosemary essential oil

Mix ingredients together, apply to face in gentle upward
strokes, rinse with luke warm, and follow with a toner
good for all skin types. Stored in refrigerator will keep
about one week or so. Full of vitamins and AHA
antioxidants. Restores a youthful glow, and smoothes fine
lines and tones, you will love it!

Chosen

Holy separate set apart for you,
sanctified chosen my Lord is it true?
Oh Holy Ghost, my comforting friend
teaching me helping me patience to the end
my ear must carefully listen to you
following instructions faithful to do
My Lord
what could you possibility see in me?
my name you called in time for choosing
Oh thank you father, for the life you give
is more than enough
so glad I've been chosen!

You have not chosen me but I have chosen you and
ordained you that you should go and bring forth
fruit, and that your fruit should remain: that
whatever you shall ask of the Father in my name,
he may give it you..

John 15 16

Cucumber wash

One puree cucumber
One tablespoon soapwort root
One tablespoon vegetable glycerin
½ tablespoon aloe vera gel
½ tablespoon of your choice of clay
One cup of water

Place soapwort root in pan with water
Slowly bring to boil, simmer about 20 minutes
Remove from heat and cool, separate soapwort from
water. Add all ingredients together, allow product to set a
little before using, about 15 minutes

Apply to damp face working up lather. A very refreshing
wash good for the entire body, add a little mint sometimes
it's great⬚

Therefore I urge you brethren in view of GOD's
mercy, to offer your bodies as living sacrifices holy
and pleasing to GOD

Romans 12

Pleasant surprise wash

One tablespoon Sour cream
One teaspoon wheat flour
One teaspoon aloe vera gel
Two or three drops of lavender an essential oil

Mix all ingredient together apply to face in slow upward circular motions, rinse clean apply toner, for all skin types.

I took a break from school to volunteer in the mission fields one of the girls was using this wash, it's great for my combination skin, and though I am back home for a while I still make and use my wash it's the best! It keeps my face clear and soft, I know exactly what's in it and I save a lot of money. And dehydrated milk can be use instead of sour cream.

Honey wash makes about 8 ounce

One tablespoon raw honey
½ teaspoon fresh lime juice
½ teaspoon tea tree essential oil

Mix all ingredients together massage into face in gentle upward motions, for oily skin
Sent in by one of the sisters in her mission in Indonesia, she says she doesn't have acne because of this wash.

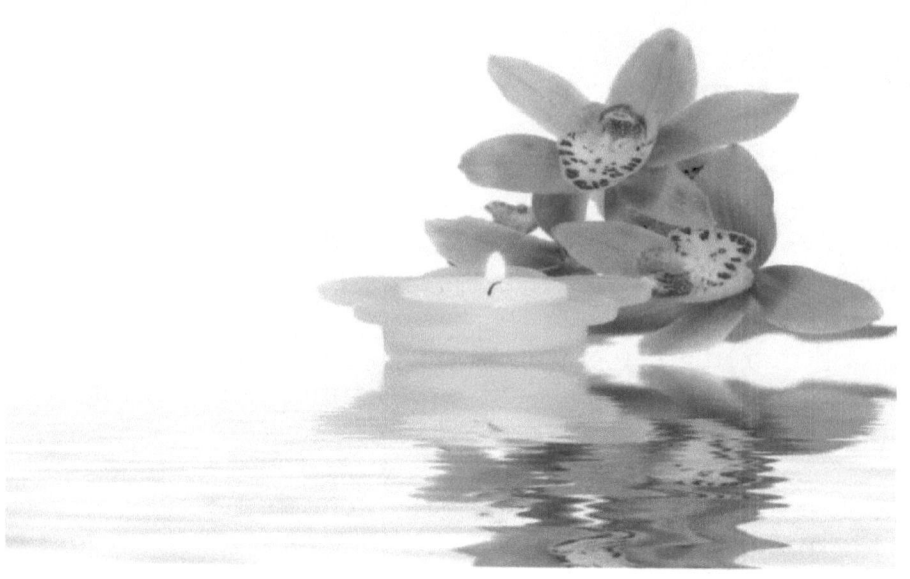

Sweet talking with Jesus
Where love freely blows
Spending time with Father Son and
Holy Ghost
Hearing his voice speak to me
Oh my GOD prayer time is so sweet.

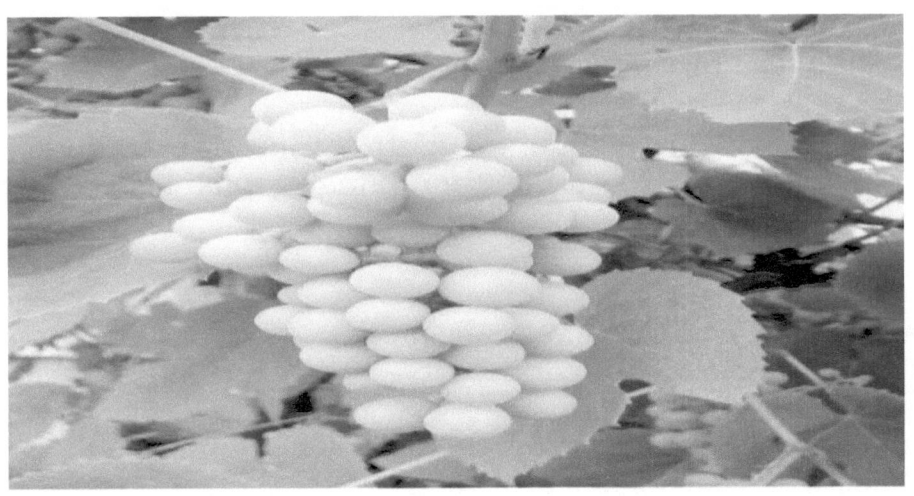

ALL NATURAL TONER'S

All skin types should use a good toner. Toners or astringents are used to aid in removing any left traces of your cleanser, and to hydrate tone and or close pores. Toners are good, so try not to skip this step. When deciding on a toner, avoid the ones that have alcohol listed in the ingredients even if you have oily skin. Here are a few toners you can create at home.

Cucumber toner,

This wonderful refreshing tonic is a terrific pick me up for your skin. It is also excellent for reducing enlarged pores, for all skin types.

Peel and Puree ½ of a cucumber
Add ½ on carbonated mineral water
Two teaspoons of apricot oil

Apply to face with a cotton ball, leave on 10 minutes.
Rinse with cool splashes of water.
Stored the rest of the tonic in a glass container and refrigerate, it will keep for about one week.
Use any time to help tone or simply to refresh tired skin.
This is the girl's favorite toner, as it helps to tone skin and tighten pores.

Witch hazel toner,

Astringent for oily and combination skin,

¼ brew cup chamomile tea
¼ cup of witch hazel,
½ tablespoon vegetable glycerin
½ tablespoon aloe vera gel
One teaspoon fresh lemon or lime juice

Brew tea first, set aside to cool
Combine all ingredients in a glass container to keep.
Shaking well before each use, apply with cotton ball, or
place ingredients in glass spray bottle shaking before use
and mist face after cleansing or anytime during the day.

Many of the Sisters use this toner and it really helps to
keep my skin clear, I shared it with some of the
missionaries in another group and they also love it also,
we're acne free.

Apple cider vinegar tonic,

This tonic is excellent for **normal and oily skin** types. Apple cider will help keep your skin healthy. The acid in the cider will aid in fighting off pimples and blemishes.

½ cup distilled water
One tablespoon apple cider vinegar
One tablespoon aloe vera gel
Two drops geranium essential oil

Combine ingredients in sterile glass container. Apply with cotton ball, shaking before each use, refrigerate. That good ole apple cider we don't leave home without it, smile!

GOD loves you no matter what may come your way
GOD loves you, stay close to him everyday!

Carrot toner,

This is a wonderful toner, excellent for **dry sensitive skin**
Carrots are full of antioxidants ready to nourish and
bless your beautiful skin with just what it needs. This
toner will tighten pores and restore a glow to skin,
nourishes, tones, and fade wrinkles.

½ cup fresh carrot juice
Two teaspoons vitamin E oil 400ui
One teaspoon wheat grass juice
½ teaspoon orange blossom oil

Mix all together, shaking before each use

Apply to face using cotton ball, let dry rinse with warm
water follow with cool to cold splashes

Place remaining toner in sterile glass container and store
in refrigerator up to one week. This toner is excellent for
mature or sun damage skin.

Thank you Toner

A few Rosemary leaves, fresh or dry
A few Thyme leaves
Plain mineral water
Steep leaves in water to make a tea, cool place in glass
spray bottle and add
One Tablespoon aloe vera gel
A drop or two of essential citrus or rose oil

This toner is wonderful it will help to tone and restore a balance to your skin.
 I went to Africa with my student group and I notice that the mothers (missionaries) there all seem to have healthy vibrant skin, by the end of the day my skin and the other student volunteers including myself, skin looked dry and tired. So I asked one of the mothers how do they do it and she told me it's our thank you toner we all use it she said, just spritz your face with it when you can throughout the day. Now I see why the mothers call this the thank you toner, because each time I use it I say thank you. Since my returning back home I have continue to use the thank you toner and my skin looks great! Thank you (smile).

Soothing Tea toner
For **delicate dry sensitive skin**

½ cup Brew chamomile tea,
½ cup of distilled water
½ teaspoon of orange blossom essential oil
Two drops of rose oil

Let tea cool, place in glass spray bottle to use as spritz to mist face when needed. Store in refrigerator shake well before each use.
 My skin is dry and sensitive, so I keep my mist bottle with me whenever possible especially when we go to very hot climates.

Let us go toner

 Mineral water toner, a great toner you can customizes according to your skin type. Use as a pick me up and refresh face any time.

Fill your (8-0z) spritz bottle with carbonated mineral water add
One tablespoon fresh lime juice
½ teaspoon lavender
a teaspoon of tea tree oil

Spritz face after cleansing or anytime you need a pick me up. This toner is good for oily skin, this one has been past on and on for years we believe it originated from one of the sisters serving her mission in the United Kingdom

Rose water

Excellent for all skin types Place several fresh rose petals in a glass (12 0z) container fill with distilled water seal and stored for about one week shaking occasionally.
And one tablespoon vegetable glycerin and a few drops of rose essential oil. Remove pedals, keep in glass or ceramic bottle.

Rachael's toner

10 ounce of rose water
Two tablespoon of vegetable glycerin
One tablespoon aloe vera gel
A couple drops of frankincense essential oil. Shake well before using can be place in spray bottle to mist your wonderful skin anytime. We have been enjoying this one for a very long time it hydrates, tones and helps reduces signs of aging. It is so simple yet we notice how pretty our skin looks and feel after using. Name after Jacob the patriarch wife.

Buttery milk toner,

One tablespoon mineral water
Two tablespoon butter milk
½ teaspoon tea tree oil
A drop of essential rose oil

Apply toner with cotton ball
Let dry then rinse with cool splashes of water. This toner
is excellent for **dry sensitive and normal skin,** helps to
soften and restore natural oils to your skin.

Toning tomato

One tomato (small) puree
One cup carbonated mineral water
Juice from one orange
½ teaspoon rose hips oil
½ teaspoon vitamin E oil
Mix all together,
Apply with cotton ball patting over face
Let dry, rinse cool splashes for **all skin types**
This antioxidant recipe conditions and restores a youthful
glow and helps reduces signs of aging.

Green Tea toner

½ cup carbonated mineral water
½ cup brew green tea
Two tablespoon glycerin
One tablespoon pure aloe vera gel
Two or three drops of rose essential oil
Combine all ingredients together in spray bottle or glass
container shake to mix before each use
For **normal to dry skin,** mist face anytime to refresh tone
and moisten skin.

Seaweed toner, #1

1/8 cup seaweed or one tablespoon seaweed extract
(Bladder wrack)
One cup plain carbonated mineral water
One teaspoon cucumber extract
½ teaspoon spirulina powder
½ teaspoon comfrey
mint oil

Combine all adding a drop or two of mint oil, apply with
cotton ball, refrigerate after use. Helps to tone, firm and
detox skin for **normal** to **Oily skin types,** this recipe has
been around among us for years and we all enjoy it.

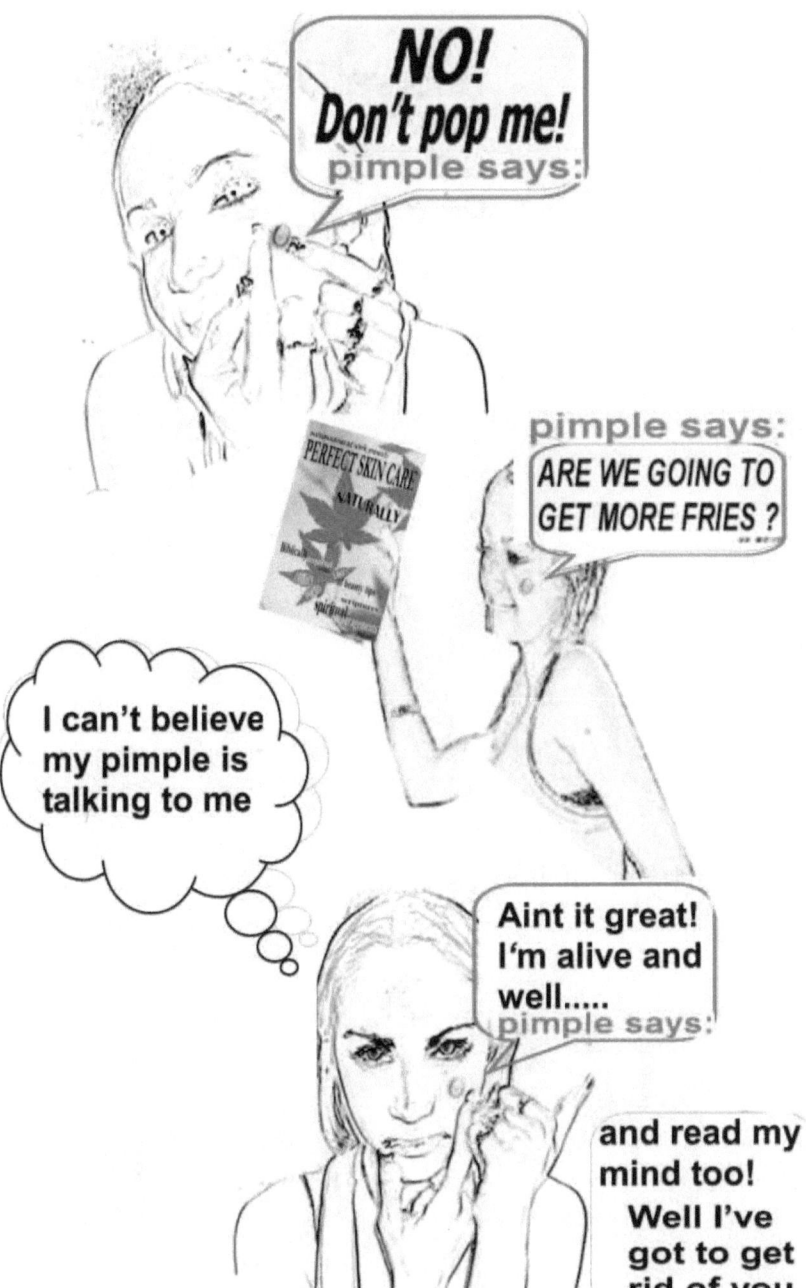

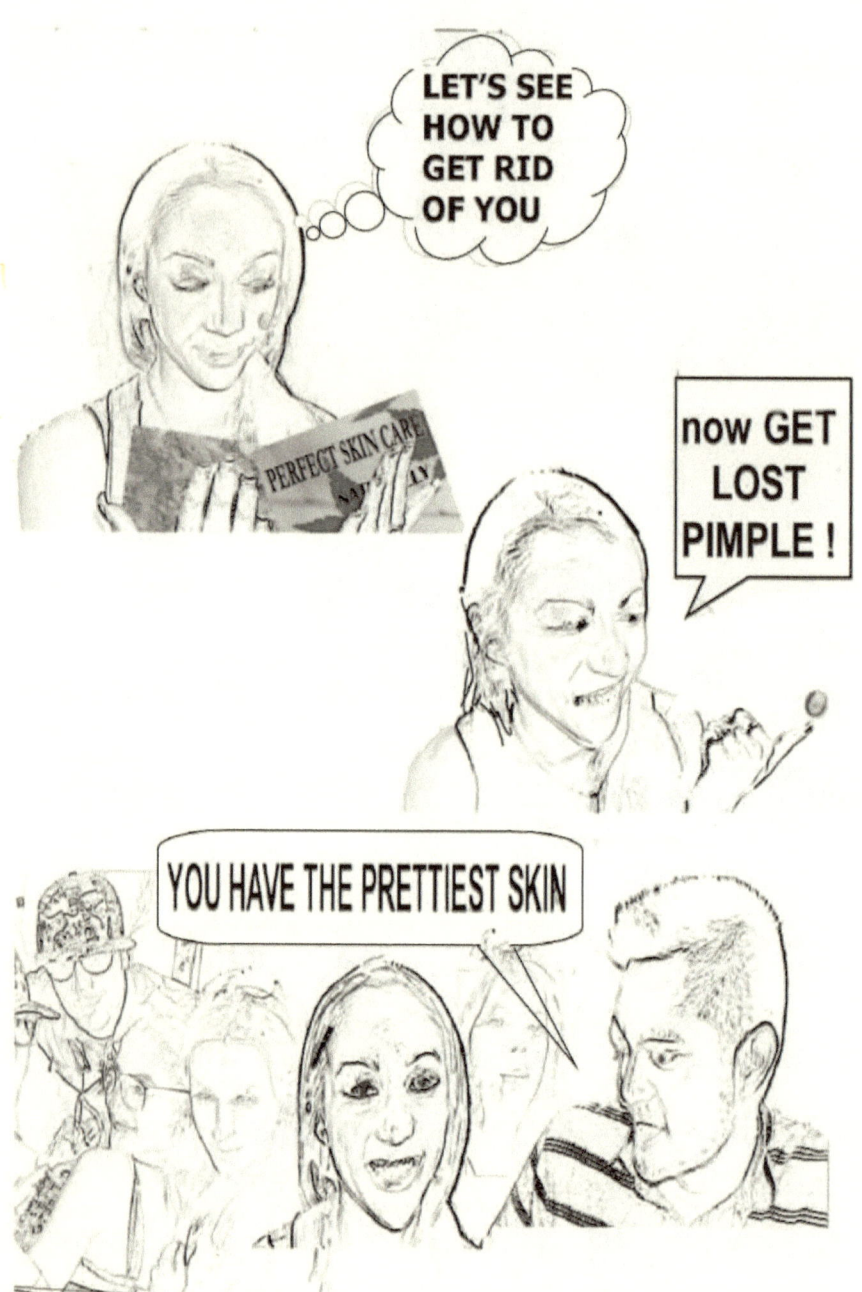

Seaweed Toner #2

¼ cup Sea weed puree or one tablespoon Sea weed extract (bladder wrack)
One-cup rose water
½ tablespoon glycerin
½ tablespoon aloe vera

A drop or two of a fragrance essential oil (your choice)
Stored in glass container and use freely
For normal to dry skin

Seaweed toners or mask's have a wonderful effect on the skin. They soften and moisten and they aid in firming and detoxifying the skin. Yet adding minerals and nutrients that are needed for the health of your skin, In addition, the high iodine content stimulates your thyroid gland increasing blood circulation, thus helping to firm and decrease any cellulite.
There are many types of sea weed. Most common is sea kelp and laminaria seaweed sheets, that are normally used for sushi rolls they may also be used for skin care.

─ ✿ ─

A

Virtuous woman

Who can find a virtuous woman?
For her price is far above Rubies

Strength and Honor
Are her clothing She openeth
her mouth and In her tongue
is the law of Kindness

She looketh well to the ways of her
House hold
Favor is deceitful and Beauty is vain

But a woman that feareth the LORD She
she shall be praise

─ ✿ ─

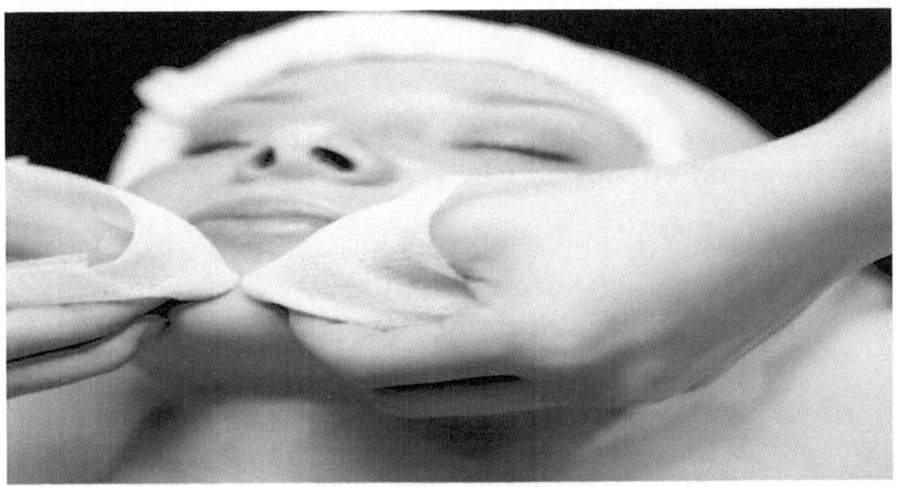

THE FACIAL

Select some time to pamper yourself...to wash your cares and stress away. A home facial can work magic to shed dead skin cells, leaving your face with a smooth, softened look. Facials are also good for increasing circulation in your face, thus helping to tone and firm, giving your face back its natural radiance. Let's begin.

A Steam Facial

A steam facial will help your pores rid themselves of impurities and encourage the growth of new skin cells.

Fill a clean bowl or basin with boiling water and add a drop or two of your favorite essential oil. Next, add a few leaves of chamomile, spearmint, rosemary or fresh thyme.

Positioning your clean face just over the bowl, about 10 inches away from the hot water, and cover both your head and the bowl with a dry towel, making a tent. Be sure not to burn yourself, nor allow steam to escape. Try to stay in this position for about 8 to 10 minutes.

Immediately follow with cool splashes of water to help close your pores and improve skin tone.

It is important to protect your open pores from air-born dust and debris, cool or cold water splashes will help close them. Also, try not to venture outdoors for at least one half hour after a steam facial.

FACIAL MASKS

A mask should always be applied to moist or damp skin, applying evenly over face and neck avoiding the delicate eye area, making sure not to pull the skin. Here are few natural masks you can create right at home; they contain many nutrients that are simply just good for your beautiful skin. Many of the girls have their favorite mask, and what a list! Enjoy!

A reminder: this is your special time you have set aside, so relax take your time.

Clays

There are several types of **clays.** Most are found at your local health food store, and some are found at the local drug store. Clay masks are rich in minerals. They work wonders. Clay masks deep clean impurities from your pores, also helping to stimulate new skin cells and tone your skin. Green and rose clay is for normal to oily skin. Blue and red clay are good for dry, sensitive skin types.

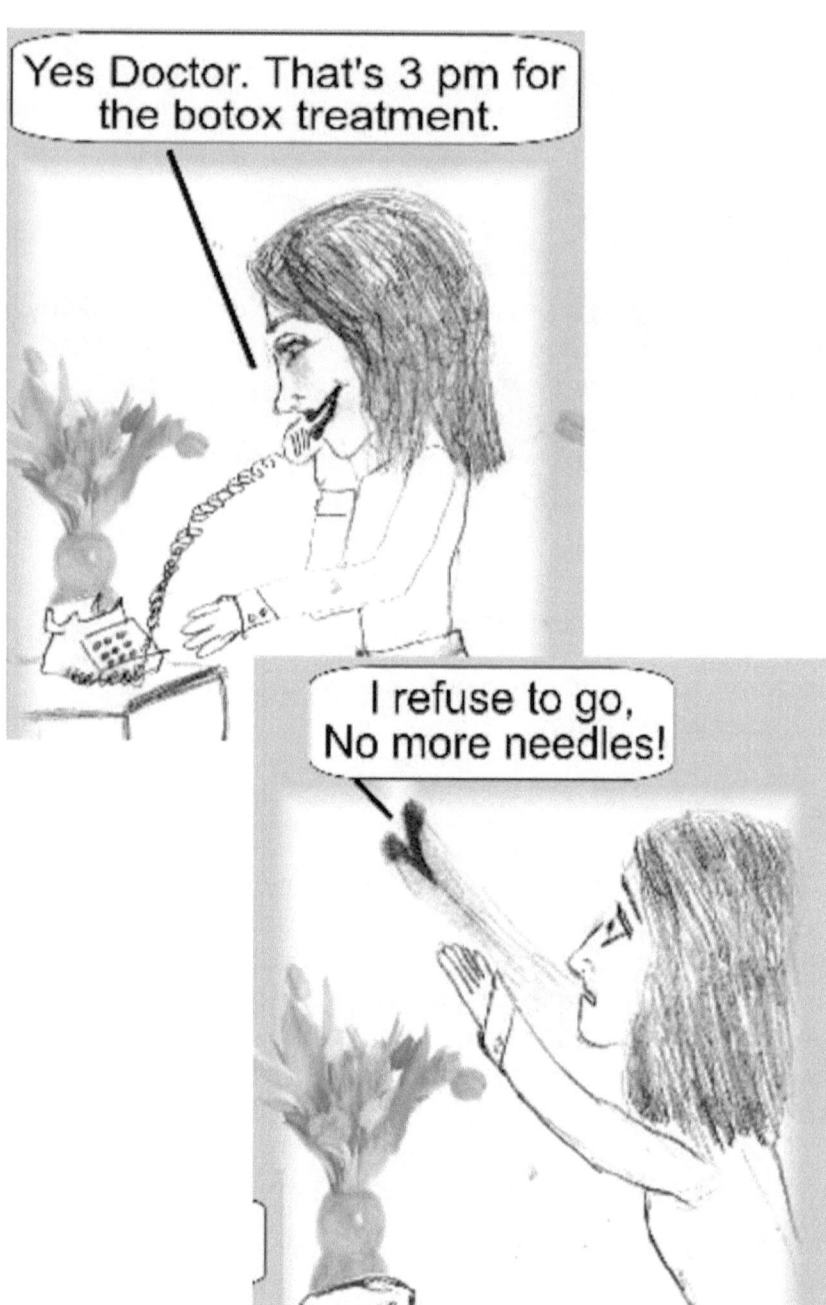

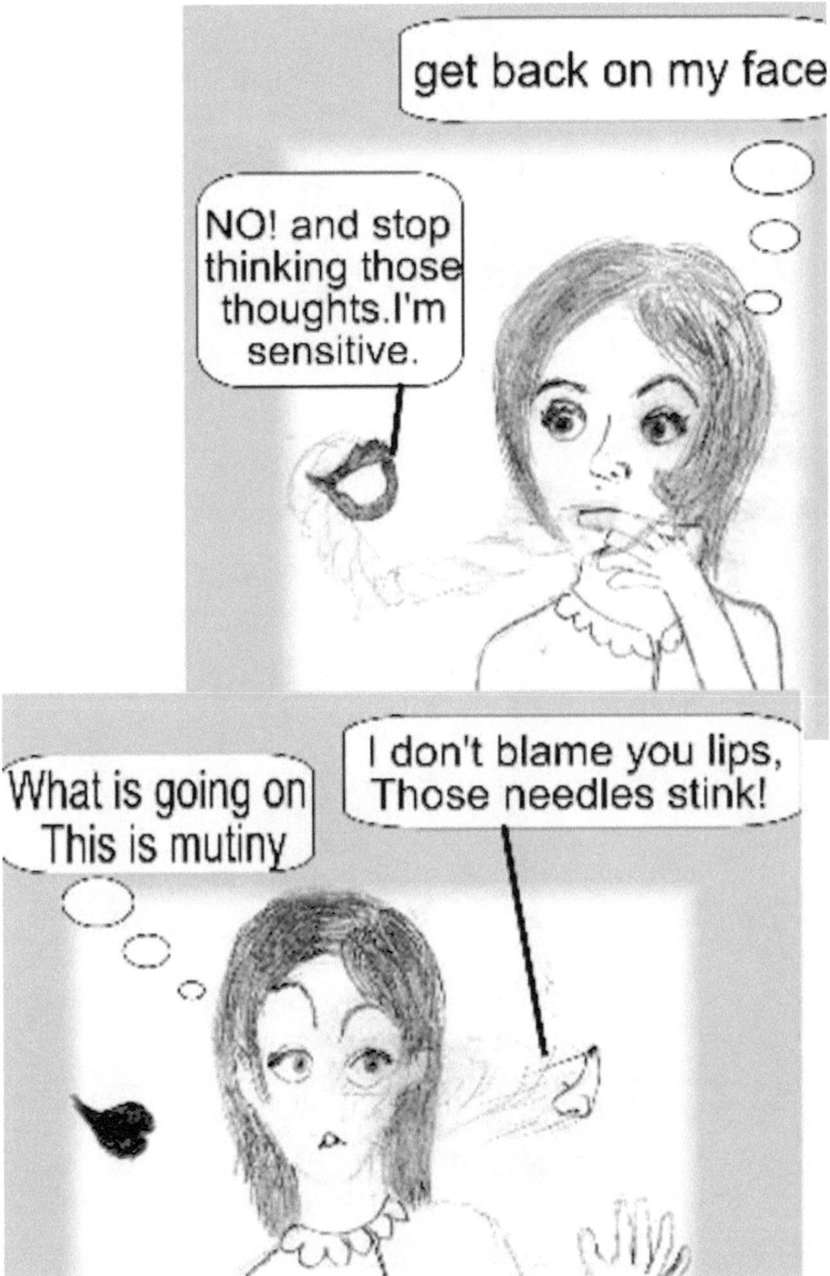

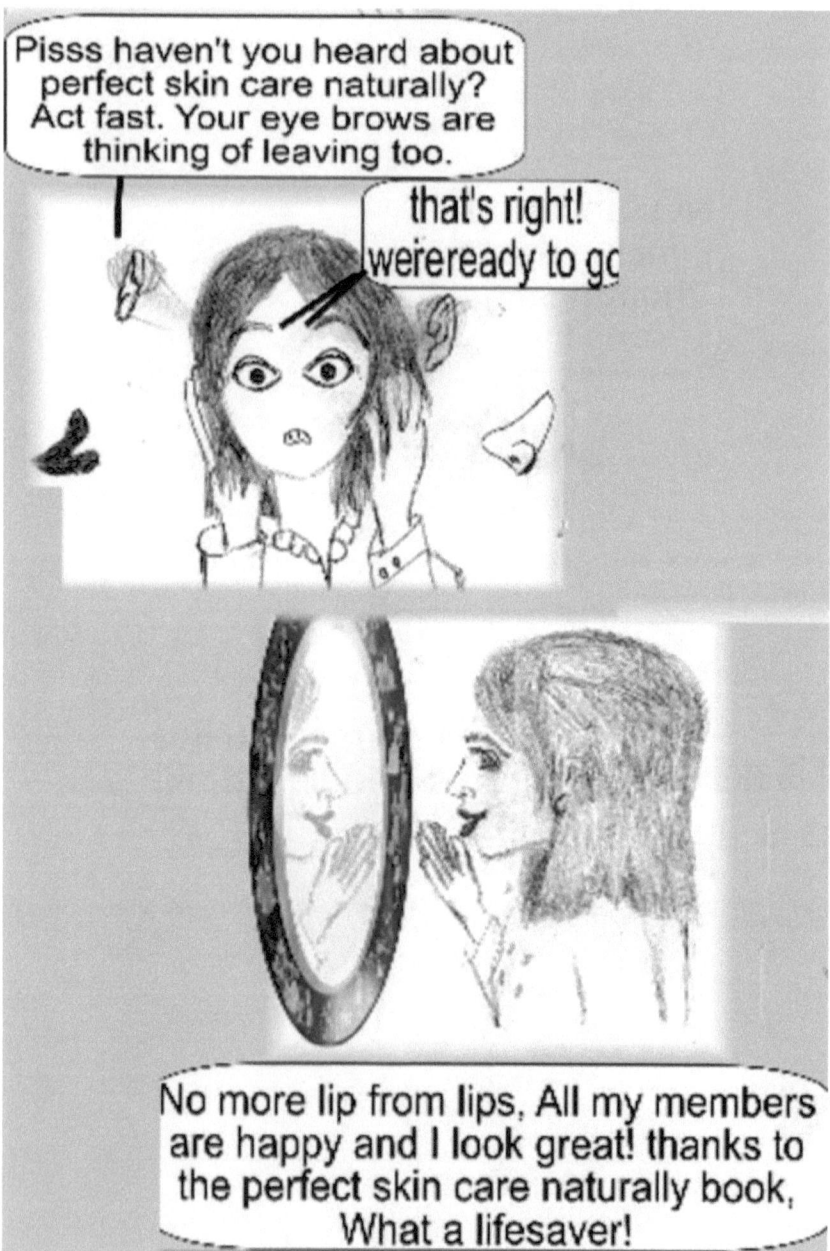

Oatmeal mask

This mask will soften and smooth skin and is excellent for all skin types acting as a natural cleanser. As the mask dries, it absorbs waste by deep cleaning your pores.

¼ cup uncooked oats
Add just enough hot mineral water or butter milk to make a soft paste, not runny whip till creamy, apply to face, 15 minutes rinse moistens and softens fine lines. This mask seems to be everyone favorite.

With my mission in Thailand every other Friday night all the girls would get together to talk and give each other facials. That was just the beginning for me since then I have always cared for my skin naturally and with my own homemade products, I love it! And my skin looks and feels great
volunteer

Moisturizing puddin mask

1/4 firm cooked oats
1/2 tablespoon or so of mayonnaise
whip w/hand mixer until creamy, warm slightly if you like, apply to clean damp, let set15 min. and rinse clean.

Avocado whip mask

 A delightful easy mask great for replenishing your beautiful skin, it is especially good for dry or normal skin types.

¼ avocado mashed
¼ teaspoon miracle whip or mayonnaise
¼ rose hips oil
Mash and mix well, apply two leave on 10 minutes, rinse clean, moisten and softens and helps prevent wrinkles.

Avocado ginseng mask

¼ avocado mashed well
½ teaspoon aloe vera gel
¼ teaspoon ginseng powder or extract

Mix and apply.
As mask starts to dry spritz with mineral water few times, leave on 20 minutes Tones and Replenishes skin with nutrients and moisture.

Avocado moisturizing mask

¼ avocado mashed
¼ cup whipped cream
¼ teaspoon carrot oil

Mix and blend all together, and apply to face, leaving on 15 minutes, rinse clean apply atoner
Helps reduce fine lines and wrinkles, and restores natural oils to skin.

Full of antioxidants, this one is so much fun to do especially with the girl friends or husband, smile.

Simple egg mask

Excellent for restoring the natural oils in your skin,
Mix one egg yolk
A teaspoon aloe vera gel

Mix, apply to face let dry, rinse off. Soften wrinkles and firm's skin, leaves face feeling and looking lifted.
This one is so easy you can give your skin a nourishing mask anytime, for dry skin.

Simply egg mask #2

Apply one egg white mix with
¼ teaspoon fresh lemon or lime juice

Let dry rinse off, helps to balance tone and lift the face.
Some of us do have oily skin but mostly it's the new girls
coming in, this mask always works wonders! For **oily to
normal** skin types.

Brewer's Yeast masque

This mask will feed your skin with vital nutrients,
Excellent for softening and reducing enlarged pores. For
all skin types

1/2 tablespoon Brewer's yeast (powder)
One tablespoon aloe vera gel
½ teaspoon Vitamin E oil

Mix, as yeast absorbs, make a soft paste,
Apply with fingertips, let dry and rinse, for normal to dry
skin. This one goes back probably 100 years or more and
we are still benefiting from it. Restores nutrients, softens
wrinkles.

Mango tropical fruit mask,

¼ cup mash mango fruit
1/8 teaspoon apricot oil (delete oil for oily skin)
1/8 teaspoon rosehip oil
Mix all, apply to face massaging ever so gently in small circular upward motions for about three minutes let rest 10 minutes, rinse.
This masque is loaded anti aging properties has vitamin C and antioxidants that renew skin and leaves it dewy soft, reducing fine lines and firming. **All skin types** will enjoy this mask.

Leah's comforting mask
(Jacob's The Patriarch wife)
Two tablespoons rose clay
One teaspoon avocado oil
½ teaspoon fresh lime juice
A drop of comfrey oil
A little mineral water, make a soft paste

Mix all and warm, apply to face leave on 10 minutes, rinse helps to de-tox skin, and refresh skin
Normal to oily skin types,

Rachel Beauty mask Jacob's (Israel wife)

Two tablespoon red clay
4 mashed berries
A little warm buttermilk, just enough to make a soft
paste, apply to entire face while still warm and let dry,
rinse warm to cool splashes leaves skin moist and dewy,
for **normal to dry skin** rich with AHA a favorite of our
many volunteers, afterwards your face really does look
more beautiful that is reason we call this one Rachel's
mask.

NOTE; when selecting the ingredients for making your
natural skin care products always strive to purchase the
most purist form of gels or clays.

Papaya fruit mask,

Take half a papaya spooning out most of the fruit. Then rub
the inside of the skin over your face and neck firmly yet
gently, leave on 10 to 15 minutes, rinse, this mask is good
for toning the skin for all skin types. Afterwards relax and
enjoy your fruit yea!

Clear skin mask

Puree a ¼ cup fresh pineapple
A little wheat flour
¼ teaspoon fresh lemon or lime juice.

Mix and apply to face, will help fight acne eruptions, leave on 10 minutes rinse clean.

Honey mask,

A great mask that deep cleans and hydrates leaving your skin dewy moist, as honey is a natural humectants retaining moisture. It is one of nature's perfect foods, it is good all by itself, add nothing. Simply apply
one tablespoon of pure raw honey to face,
leave on about 10 minutes.
Rinse warm water then cool splashes, pat dry
Good for all skin types.

Martha, Martha egg mask

One egg white
One teaspoon of honey,
One 1/8 cup cooked oats

Mix with hand mixer till creamy warm slightly and apply
to face, set 15 minutes Rinse with Luke warm water
following with cool splashes. For **all skin types** firms and
restores nutrients and moisture to skin. A simple basic
firming egg mask,

And Jesus Answered: Martha, Martha, you are worried
and upset about many things but one thing is needful
Luke 10,41

Avocado Yogurt mask

Combine ¼ mashed Avocado
½ tablespoon plain yogurt, mix creamy then using your
fingertips, apply to face leave on about 15 minutes, rinse,
pat dry, a moisturizing mask, your skin will love it! for
normal and dry skin types.

Naomi citrus mask
(book of Ruth)
¼ cup of plain yogurt and
 Wheat flour or powder oats
A drop of frankincense oil

Blend together to make a soft paste, will leave face
looking and feeling fresh and soft for **all skin types.**
We call this mask Naomi mask because after you tried the
expensive store bought jars you will come back to this
simple homemade mask. It is full of nourishment and
helps to deep clean and renew skin, you will love it.

Vitamin C mask,

One teaspoon vitamin C powder crystals
One tablespoon aloe vera gel
A drop or two of rose hip oil
A drop or two of orange blossom essential oil

Mix and apply over entire face and neck helps to smooth
out fine lines & wrinkles, good for normal and dry skin.

Sea mask

Spirulina is green algae powder, high in protein w/
vitamins A and B family, so it has just what our skin
needs, good for **all skin types**

½ tablespoon spirulina powder
One teaspoon of black currant seed oil
One teaspoon carrot oil

Apply with facial brush, let dry rinse follow with toner, a
firming masque, deep cleans and clarifies skin.

Queen Sheba firming mask

½ tablespoons of dry powder seaweed or kelp powder
½ tablespoon vegetable glycerin
½ teaspoon jojoba oil
½ teaspoon bladder wrack, extract (seaweed)

Apply to face with soft facial brush dry, rinse, excellent
for **normal to dry skin**, softens tones and detoxifies skin.

Moisturizing tropical mask

1/8 cup sour cream
One teaspoon coconut milk
½ teaspoon pineapple juice
Powder oats or wheat pastry flour (enough to make a soft paste)

Mix and mashed all ingredients together, apply to face, with facial brush leave on 15 minutes rinse, cool splashes

Replenishes skin with natural oils, and antioxidants, rich in vitamin A and C apply toner afterward,

Fruity clarifying mask

Two tablespoon rose clay
One tablespoon plain yogurt
Enough pineapple juice to make a nice paste
A drop of lemon essential oil

Apply to face, leave on 15 minutes, rinse, helps to deep clean pores and blemishes and **acne** also reduces enlarge pores.

Fresh Breeze mask

One tablespoon Brew mint tea
One tablespoon vegetable glycerin
One tablespoon pectin
One tablespoon aloe vera gel
2 drops a mint oil
Two slices of cucumber

Combine glycerin, aloe vera and tea, using your electric mixer on low speed, slowly add in pectin, the mixture will start to thicken allow to rest for about ½ hour enough for mixture to set.

Then add in the oils, the cucumbers are for your eyes, cucumbers will help tone skin and aids in fading dark circles. Apply mask evenly on face leave on about 15 minutes, rinse clean apply toner, take the time and treat your skin to this one.

O LORD let thy loving kindness and thy truth continually preserve me.
Psalm 40

Lord you're holding me

Through deep valleys and great struggles he
seen me through,
I Look at him and in his arms
I Run into

LORD, you hold me day and night and
I thank you
For you are more than wonderful to me
And far beyond all beauty I see
And you are more worthy then anyone
could ever be
Your blanket of mercy your stretch
forth arms
Your loving hands caress until dawn
My faiths in you my Lord I shout
My vision clear there is no doubt

And when life cares tried to destroy me,
I stand secure for Lord you're holding me

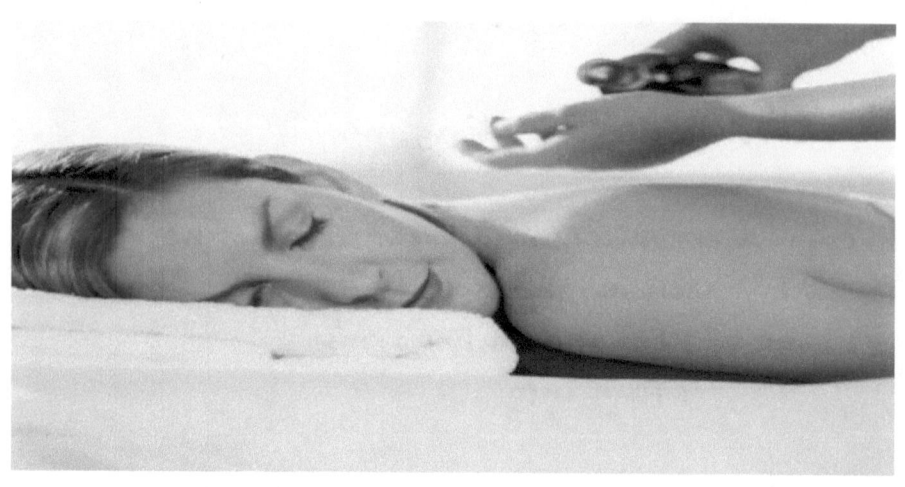

Each day is a <u>present</u> given
by GOD
unwrap your day with joy and
Great expectation!

LORD our Lord

O When I consider your heavens
The work of your fingers the moon and stars,
Which you have set in place
What is man that you are mindful of
Him, and
The son of man that you care for him

You made him a little lower then the
Angels
And hast crowned him with glory and
Honor
You made him ruler over the works of your
hands
You put everything under his feet
O LORD our Lord how majestic is your name
in All the earth

psalm 8

Banana firming mask

Mix one ½ mash banana
One tablespoon whip cream
One teaspoon aloe vera gel
A few drops of vitamin E oil

Mix well, apply to skin, massaging in slowly remove with splashes of warm to cool water
This is a fun one got to do it when you get together with friends.

Toning berry mask

3 or 4 strawberries mashed well
One tablespoon of egg whites
One tablespoon cooked oats

Apply to clean face
Let dry about 10 minutes, rinse with Luke warm water, and follow with cool water rinsing. Tones and condition skin for oily skin.

Ruth moisturizing mask

1 tbsp regular plain yogurt
1 tbsp cooked oats
Two teaspoon extra virgin olive oil

Mix well together then apply to clean face, let set, about ten minutes. Rinse with Luke water, following with cool splashes. Helps replenish moisture and reduce signs of aging skin, with anti aging nutrients, A gentle moisturizing mask, so many of the girls say this one is the best, enjoy!

Book of Ruth: for where you go I will go and where you stay I will stay thy people shall be my people, and thy God my God, said Ruth. Ruth 1, 16

Rebekah beauty mask

1 tbsp cooked oats,
1 tbsp aloe vera gel
1 tbsp egg white
A drop each of frankincense & myrrh

Mix warm and apply to face, let set, rinse w/Luke water and cool splashes following, pat dry,
For normal to combination skin, helps to tone and firms skin . This mask was inspired by the tales of Rebekah, Isaac's wife (book of Genesis).

Clear skin Mask

1 tbsp regular plain yogurt
1 tsp lemon or lime juice
1 tsp wheat flour
Mix, apply to skin, let set about 10-15 minutes
Rinse Luke water, pat dry for **oily skin use twice a week.** A lot of the young volunteers say this is the best, and we believe it! Their skin is soft and clear, the acne is all gone!

Natural Peel

You can exfoliate your skin before using this peel.

Two teaspoons aloe vera gel
¼ teaspoon fruit extract
A drop of citrus essential oil

Mix and apply to face, let set, then rinse, follow with toner and moisturizer.

Zipporah Ethiopian mask

½ tbsp puree cucumber
¼ avocado mashed
½ tbsp cooked oats
A teaspoon aloe vera gel
Two drops of mint extract

Combine all apply to skin let set about 15 minutes, rinse clean excellent toning and firming mask, for normal to **dry skin n**amed after Moses wife,

I want to be gorgeous!

I want a be gorgeous all the days long,
I want a sock it to the fellows though I'll do
no
Wrong
No I'm not like those others with naughty ways
And all
just want to be gorgeous all my years long!

Egyptian mask

Puree ¼ of an apple,
One teaspoon wheat grass juice
One teaspoon aloe vera juice
½ teaspoon wheat flour
A little fresh lime juice

Mix all together, apply to face, relax keep on 15 to 20
minutes, cored apple to puree but leave skin on **normal
to oily skin**, This mask helps to rejuvenate your skin.
Full of nutrients your skin will drink up and love, reveals
a fresh new glow..

Earth mask

Two tablespoons red clay
One teaspoon, honey
One teaspoon extra virgin olive oil
One egg yolk
Drop of frankincense

Mix together, warm slightly apply, and leave on until dry
Rinse clean, apply toner, a moisturizing masque reducing
signs of aging, smooth's wrinkles.

Queen Esther beauty mask

One egg yolk
¼ cup cooked oats
One tablespoon plain yogurt
½ teaspoon vitamin E oil
A drop of frankincense

Warm and mix together to make a soft paste
Apply relax let dry about 15 minutes rinse clean with
cool splashes. This is a lovely mask treat yourself to it.

Take me away mask

2 mashed strawberries
1/8 cup of whipping cream
¼ cup cooked oats
One teaspoon aloe vera gel

Mix, warm slightly in micro-wave apply to skin leave on
10 minutes. Refreshing moisturizing mask, this is a very
special mask go ahead and treat your skin to it.

Easy Seaweed masque

You will need Seaweed
A Steam towel
Warm mineral water
And fresh lime juice

A few sheets of sea weed. (sushi rolls)
Place the seaweed in warm mineral water with lime juice
to soak about 5 minutes, remove seaweed and place towel
in water and warm in micro wave.
Then apply sheets to face leaving an opening for the nose

Place warm steam towel over sheets and face
Leave on 10 minutes,

This mask will help to deep clean your pores and will
encourage skin cell renewal. The seaweed will draw out
impurities fro your skin. It also helps to reduce cellulite if
applied over body areas where there is cellulite. This
mask will help detox the skin and fight acne. Follow with
a toner or astringent.

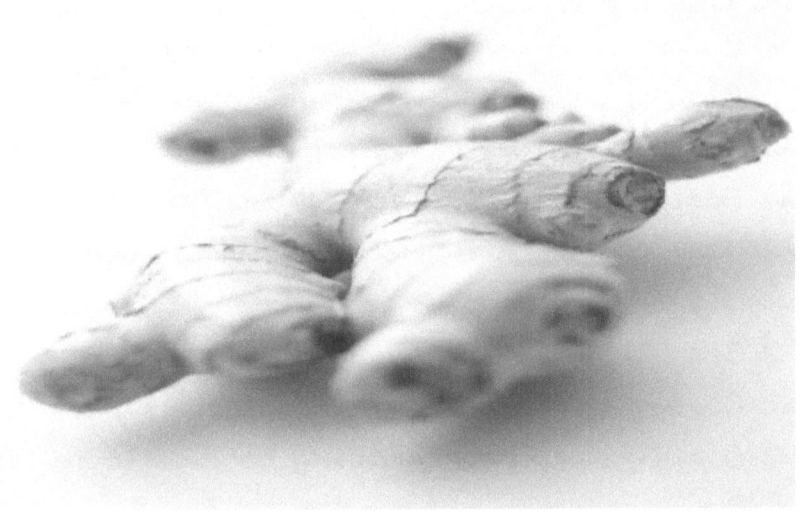

The recipes measurements are normally for one
application for face but all masks maybe applied to the
entire body, avoiding the genital area is a good idea.
When doing a body mask just make more of the product
of course.
Exfoliate your body in the shower, and while skin is damp
apply mask. Lying down covering yourself with a large
warm towel, or plastic sheet about 15 minutes, then
rinsing clean in the shower
Give your beautiful skin a treatment it deserves.

The Beauty Within

The Beauty within is, the love you feel

The Beauty within is, when you consider others

The Beauty within is, protecting the defenseless

The Beauty within is, being thankful

The Beauty within is, Helping giving and sharing

The Beauty within is, enjoying life

The Beauty within is, respecting your elders

The Beauty within is, praying for and loving the young

The Beauty within is, knowing your specially made for a purpose

The Beauty within is, receiving the Holy Ghost and letting him lead you to complete your purpose

the Beauty within is, the fruits of the Spirit which is Love, joy, peace ,patience, gentleness, goodness faith, meekness, and self control against such there is no law

The Beauty within is your conscience

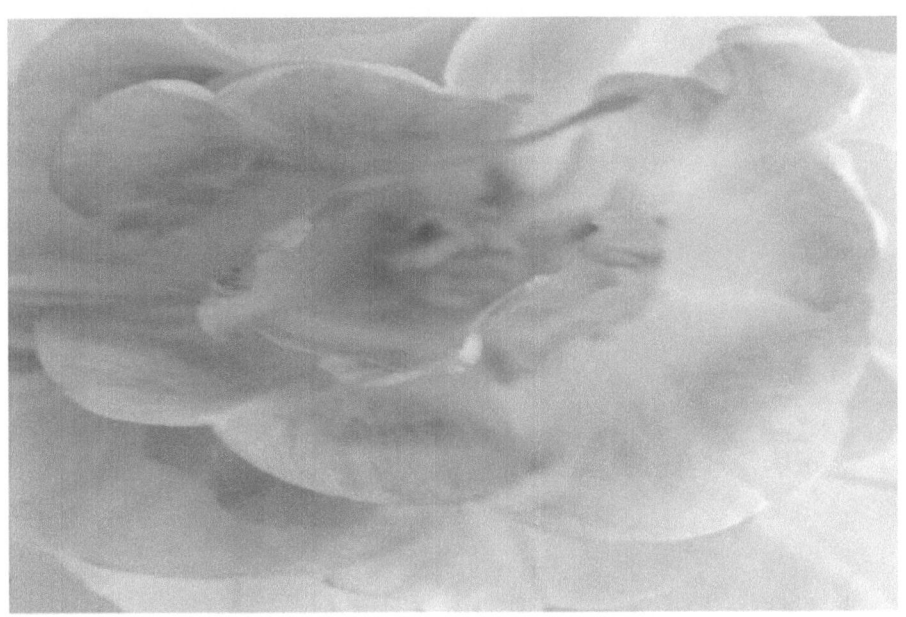

He had made everything
       Beautiful In its time

Ecclesiastes 3:11

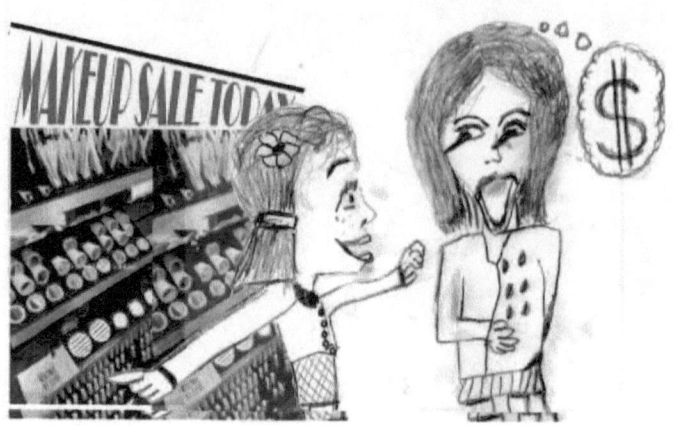

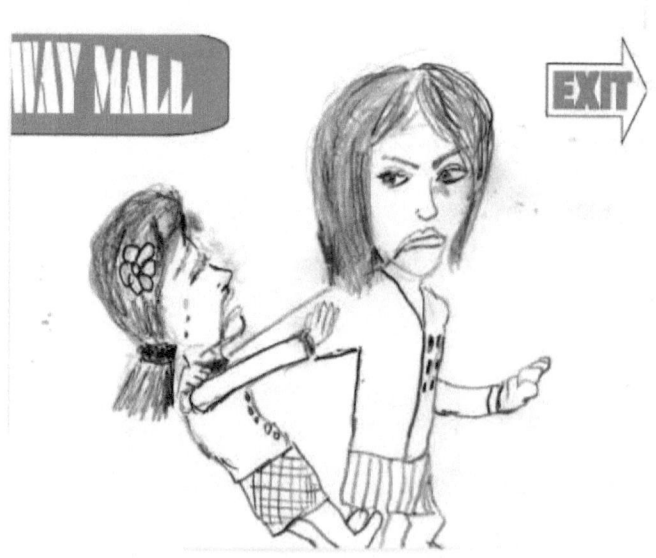

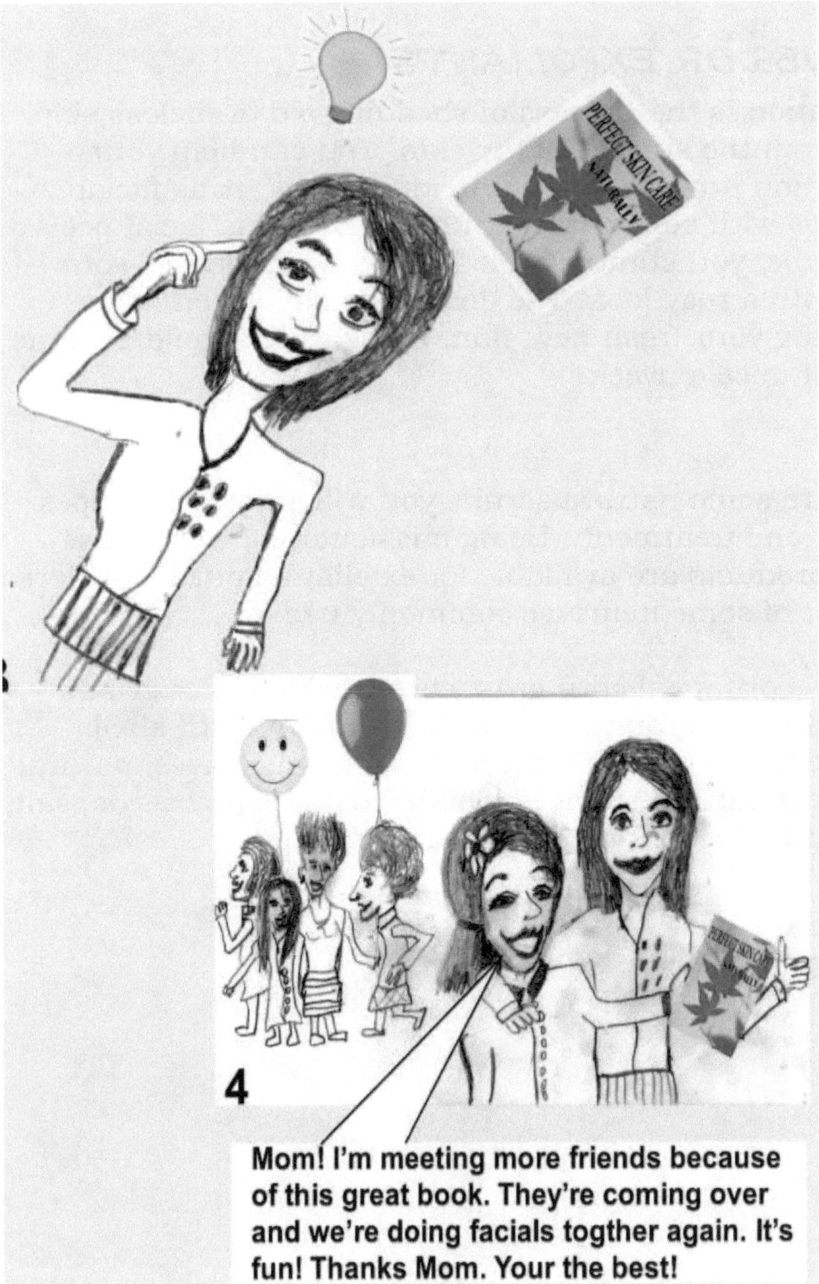

Mom! I'm meeting more friends because of this great book. They're coming over and we're doing facials togther again. It's fun! Thanks Mom. Your the best!

SCRUBS OR EXFOLIANT'S

Exfoliation is the process of shedding old or lifeless skin cells from the surface of the skin. You can help your exfoliation process move more quickly by using facial brushes with soft, natural bristles. By using facial peels or scrubs, you stimulate blood flow, which leaves your skin with a rosy look. The dead cells have been lifted, revealing your fresh new skin. Exfoliating should be done at least once a week.

Here are some natural scrubs you will enjoy. All recipes are for one treatment. Being missionaries, we will use what products are available for exfoliating our skin. Here is a list of some items we commonly use:

Berries,corn meal,corn grits, corn husks, coffee grinds ground sand, ground tree bark, ground walnut shells ground barley, uncooked grounded beans leaves, natural brushes, natural sponges loofahs, oats, poppy seeds, salt, ground fruit seeds sugar, wheat germ.

Dry Brush Massage

This wonderful beauty treatment has health benefits also. Dry brush massaging will improve your blood circulation and will help your body to rid itself of toxins and impurities. The brushing removes layers of dead skin revealing the younger looking and softer feeling skin. In addition dry brush massaging aids in breaking up cellulite.

It is important to use a brush made of natural bristles, not of nylon or synthetic man made products. Synthetic products can damage your skin, so natural bristles are best. Apply eucalyptus or tea tree essential oil on the brush bristles and begin. Start the massage at the feet brushing vigorously upward in circular motions. Don't forget you back and arms pits, as well as the palm of your hands. Make sure to brush vigorously, yet gently, stroking upward towards the heart. This process is very stimulating.

Continue brushing your sweet skin for a few minutes, then rinse in the shower. After this treatment skin will feel toned and refreshed; it's simply great!

Take care of your **brush** or **loofah**. After each use, shake out any dead skin flakes that may have gotten caught in your brush. Then rinse, and place it in the sun to help naturally cleanse it of bacteria, which can build up.

Pilgrim facial scrub,

1/2 teaspoon cooked oats
1/2 teaspoon ground corn meal
Two teaspoons sweet almond oil
1/4 teaspoon chamomile extract

Mix, making a paste apply to face and neck massaging
gently in upward circular motions, rinse, leaves skin fresh
and dewy helps remove dead skin cells.
Apply toner, use moisturizer if skin is dry.

Strawberry polish

Two or three mashed strawberries
One tablespoons plain yogurt
One tablespoon finely ground almonds

Mix together, massage into skin rinse luke warm water
then cool splashes leave's your skin rejuvenated with AHA
nourishment.
For all skin types add a few drops two of Almond oil if
you like for a soft refresh look.

Miriam facial scrub

A teaspoon finely ground kosher salt
A teaspoon raw honey
½ teaspoon almond oil
½ teaspoon wheat germ oil
A drop of vanilla oil
A drop of mint oil

Combine ingredients, then massage gently to exfoliate, rinse pat dry apply toner, refreshing scrub,

For many years several of the sisters have used this one as a body scrub it is a definite favorite. For all skin types, inspired by the story of Miriam, Moses sister.

Solid ground

When my day is up I think of you

how you fill my heart with gladness
When my day is down I think of you

and you take away my sadness

No matter what may come my way I
expect to win in him each day Whether

my day is up or down Lord you are my

Solid ground!

Galilee Sea Scrub

¼ teaspoon finely ground kosher salt
¼ mashed avocado
½teaspoon sesame or grape seed oil
A drop of myrrh oil

Mix together apply to skin remember massage gently in circular motions, rinse clean, and apply toner. This moisturizing scrub has been passed around among us since before any of us can remember. One of the sisters bought it back from her mission in Israel.

Love I saw you walking down the road
you were walking fast
      now you're walking slow,
where are you going today?

    Everywhere, when we Pray!

Ethiopian scrub

One teaspoon finely ground almonds
1 teaspoon almond meal
1 teaspoon yogurt
Two teaspoons sesame oil
A drop of orange blossom oil
A drop of mint extracts

Mix, and apply rubbing gently into skin in small circular motion to exfoliate the skin and reveal the fresh youthful skin beneath it. Rinse clean, for normal to dry skin, fill with antioxidants, great for skin renewal.

Honey mask scrub

½ tablespoon pure honey
½ teaspoon sugar
Teaspoon macadamia oil

Mix together and warm slightly massage in gentle upward strokes for a minute or two rinse clean, helps to smooth out wrinkles, cleanses and exfoliate and hydrates in one-step its great!

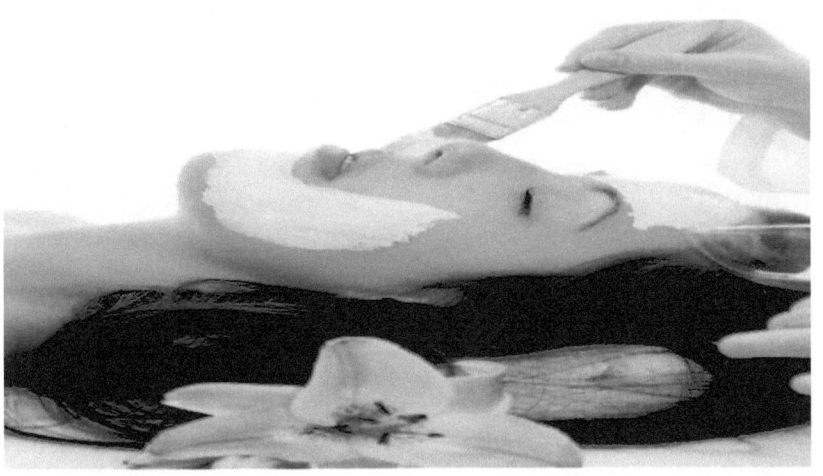

Love is
    When the boy calls
        Love is
    When he pays for dinner
        Love is
When he does not, expect me to
        fornicate!

Ginger Butter scrub

1/8 cup sugar
¼-cup soft butter
a teaspoon corn starch
½ teaspoon orange peels
½ teaspoon tea tree oil
½ teaspoon ginger extract
Drop of lemon essential oil

Mix apply gently to skin, a fun vigorous refreshing scrub
for **all skin types**. Leaves skin soft and moist, you will
love this one just as we do.

Rose body scrub

2 cups whip cream
½ cup ground almond powder or ground oats
One tablespoons raw honey
One tablespoons sweet almond oil
A few drops of rose oil
2 drops of chamomile essential oil

Gently rub in circular motions entire
body while in shower or bath.
Rinse and pat dry, cleans and soften skin, treat your skin
to this one, it's fun!

Rich moisturizing scrub

One-tablespoon sour cream
½-teaspoon finely ground kosher salt
One-teaspoon mashed avocado

Combine all ingredients, apply to skin rubbing gently, rinse with warm water follow with cool splashes of mineral water, for all skin types. This one is so easy and it is one of the best scrubs. Cleans hydrates and softens skin, enjoy!

Papaya scrub

¼ mashed papaya
½-teaspoon ground vitamin C crystals
A teaspoon aloe vera gel
1/8 teaspoon fresh crush thyme
½ teaspoon sweet almond oil

Mix all ingredients; apply to skin, a moisturizing scrub. Softens and helps to prevent wrinkles, replenishes skin with lots of anti-aging antioxidants. For normal to oily skin, be Bless! Enjoy it.

Borax
Is a white crystalline mineral salt with an alkaline taste. Used as a flux, to help blend the natural ingredients together for our hand creams and lotions.

Bee wax
Bee's secrete this and use for building their Honeycombs.

Vegetable wax, (emulsifying)
Vegetable wax is the wax that is found on the leaves of fruit trees, stems and most plants.

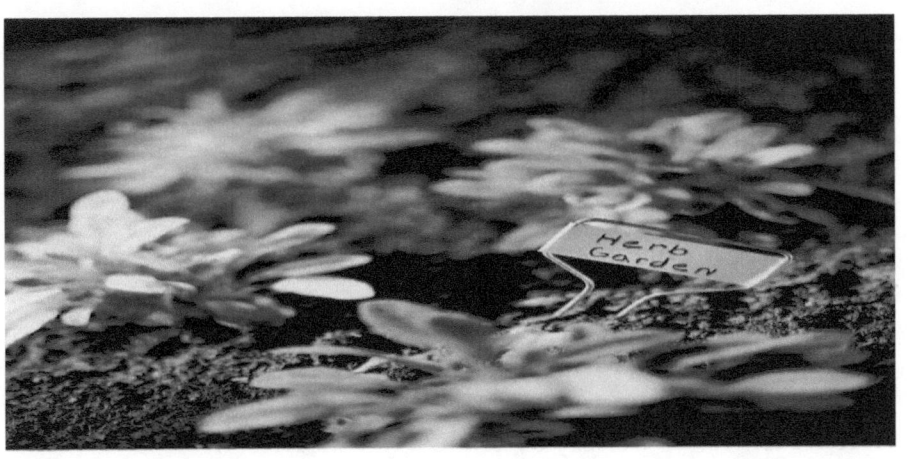

A little help from here and there ...
a little pretty a little care ...
makes one beauty beyond compare
with a little help from here and there

Basic Skin Cream makes about 2. oz

¼ cup plain mineral water
One heaping tablespoon vitamin E Oil
One tablespoon beeswax
¼ teaspoon borax
A drop or two of rose essential oil

Place beeswax and vitamin E Oil in double boiler or sauce pan on low temperature to melt
Warm mineral water, and slowly stir into melted beeswax mixture from heat and slowly mix in borax until thick and creamy, add rose oil. Place in container and refrigerate until ready to use. This is our basic recipe for skin cream, it can be customize according to your skin type so be sure to experiment, by adding vitamins, oils or fragrances and have fun!

You can add additional natural ingredients to met your skin care needs.

Basic face cream #2 makes about 2.0z

¼ cup mineral water
One teaspoon witch hazel or fresh lime juice
Two teaspoons vegetable glycerin
Two teaspoon tea tree oil
One tablespoon vegetable wax
¼ teaspoon borax
A few drops lavender essential oil

Place vegetable wax and tea tree oil in double boiler or saucepan on low temperature. Warm mineral water, witch hazel, and vegetable glycerin together stir with wooden spoon until blended. Remove from heat, slowly add water mixture to melted wax, and blend on low speed add the borax mix until thicken and creamy. Add lavender oil and refrigerate until ready to use. For oily skin, but remember try to experiment Customize your skin care Products. Try substituting fresh cucumber juice or tea for the water.

Basic face cream #3

¼ cup warm mineral
One Tablespoon aloe vera gel
1/2 Tablespoon beeswax
2 teaspoons sweet almond oil
One teaspoon lanolin
¼ teaspoon borax
 A drop or two of orange blossom essential oil
Melt almond oil, beeswax and lanolin together in double
boiler on a low temperature
Stir in warm water and aloe vera, Add to melted wax
mixture, remove from heat, blend in on low speed borax
until thick and creamy, add orange blossom oil,
refrigerate until ready to use. For dry skin, it is so
satisfying to make your own skin produces why not add
in extra antioxidants or vitamins, it wouldn't hurt.

Basic lotion

1/2 cup mineral water
A tablespoon vegetable emulsifying wax
One tablespoon aloe vera gel
One tablespoon avocado oil
One teaspoon lanolin
¼ teaspoon borax
A couple drop lavender essential oil
A couple drop carrot seed oil

Melt wax, oil, and lanolin together in double boiler or saucepan on low temperature heat water and glycerin blend with wooden spoon and add to
wax mixture. Blend in slowly with mixer the borax. This is our basic lotion recipe experiment by adding
different oils, fragrances and extracts, according to your skin type. makes about 8 ounces

moisturizing oil blend

One tablespoon vegetable glycerin
One tablespoon aloe vera
One teaspoon avocado oil
One teaspoon rose hip oil
One teaspoon sweet almond oil
One teaspoon jojoba oil
A couple drops rose oil
One cinnamon stick

Mix together and stored for a day before using. Try fruit
extracts with orange or lemon peels, let your mind
explore the herbs like thyme or rosemary instead of the
cinnamon if you will like. For all skin types, makes about
half a cup Increase the ingredients and make a nice batch
up and place in a decorative glass bottles and offer them
as gifts.

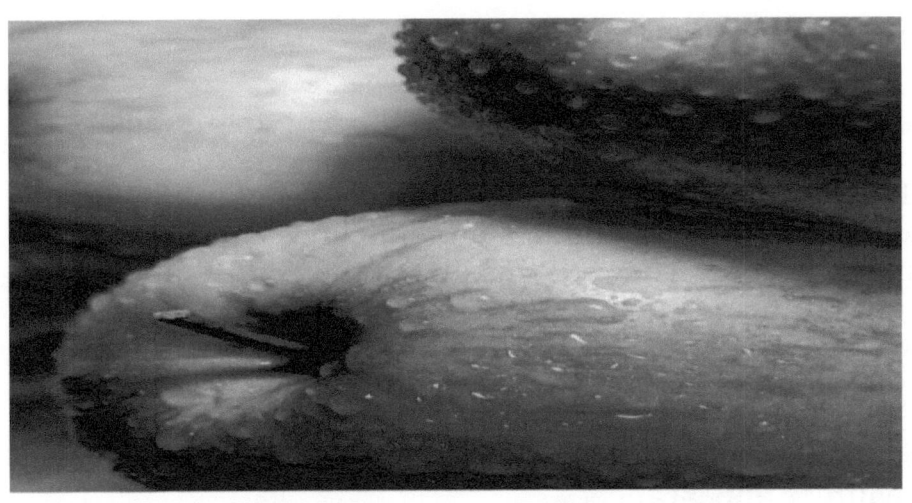

The fragrances of your breath is like
apples,
Your lips
drop sweetness as the
honeycomb my bride
Milk and honey are under your
tongue you are a garden locked up my
sister My Bride you are a spring
enclosed, a   Sealed fountain.

Song of Solomon

Facial exercises

Many of us have been somewhat diligent about facial exercising, and have truly seen the difference. Knowing that your muscles can be developed, sagging skin can be toned and firmed; wrinkles and fine lines can be smoothed out. Knowing this leaves the control knob in your hands. Focusing on exercising your facial muscles will inspire them to strengthen, thus firming and toning your skin. You can restore or maintain elasticity and a vibrant glow. Facial exercises will help do this. Your blood circulation will increase throughout the face giving you a healthier appearance.

The first thing is to pick a good time to exercise, preferably right before bedtime. The exercises will help you to relax and your face will look more vibrant in the morning.

After pinning you hair back from your face and applying a rich moisturizer to your clean face, look into the mirror. If you are interested in maintaining your youthful appearance you will need to make a commitment to do facial exercises two or three times a week as preventative maintenance. On the other hand, if you are interested in restoring and firming you should do your exercises everyday and for faster results, twice a day.

Remembering it will take a little time before seeing any results, but you should be able to feel it right away. And you will be ever so glad you did begin a facial exercise routine.

Facial exercise #1

This exercise will help tone the mouth and jaw area and smooth out smile lines. With your facial muscle
1. Pull your lips back as far as possible to make a sneer yet baring your teeth
2. Hold in that position count to 15... Relax
3. Repeat 10 times
This exercise will help smooth out you smile lines and firm and tone your jaw area, by strengthen the muscle in that area.

Facial exercise #2

This exercise will help to tone the chin and neck muscles.
1. Place your elbow on a firm place (desktop)
2. Resting your chin in the heel of your palm (the palm of
   the elbow that is resting on the desktop)
   try to open your mouth by pushing against the heel of
   your palm being sure to resist with your hand.
   pressing against the resistance
3. Relax
4. Repeat 10 times

This resistance exercise helps to fight a sagging chin or
the dreaded turkey neck.

Facial exercise #3
This exercise is to smooth out smile lines.

1. Inhaling through the nose enough air to fill up your
   Lungs.
2. Forming your lips to a whistle position
3. Filling your cheeks with the air in your lungs making
sure not to let the air escape out through your lips
4. Hold for the count of five
5. Exhale the air through your whistle shaped lips
6. Relax
7. Repeat seven times.

Facial exercise #4

1. letting the jaw hang loose, but keeping the mouth closed, the mouth area should remain relax with no tension.
2. Moving only the corners of your mouth raising them slowly upward as far as they will go.
3. staying relaxed, being careful not to crinkle your forehead
4. Relax
5. Repeat exercise 15 times

This exercise is done very slowly with direct controlled movements your consistency will pay off in time, tones facial muscles.

Therefore as God's chosen people holy and dearly loved clothe yourselves with compassion, kindness, humility, gentleness and patience. Colossian 3 12

Facial exercise #5

This exercise will help tuck your jaw area
1. Tilting your head back as far as it will go
2. Your mouth should be slightly open, not revealing your teeth.
3. Extending your jaw outward as far as it will go forming an extreme under bite.
4. Opening and closing your jaw in a chewing motion, as you move your jaws your lips should touch slightly
5. Chewing in this position 10 times.
6. Relax bring your head forward to rest
7. Repeat 5 times gradually increasing.

And whatsoever you do, work at it with all your heart as working for the Lord and not for men since you know you will receive an inheritance from the Lord as a reward. It is the Lord Christ you are serving.

Colossians 3 24

Facial exercise #6

This exercise will help smooth lines in forehead, and will help strengthen the eye brow muscles to give your face at lift.
1. place your middle fingers over your eyebrow to prevent them from rising
2. now lift the forehead muscles up and down making sure
     not to wrinkle the forehead skin.
3. Relax your forehead but keep your fingers over your eyebrows.
4. Repeat exercise eight times

Facial exercise #7

This exercise helps to tone the chin area,
with the back of your hand simply slap under your chin firmly and quickly about 50 times.
This easy exercise will help stimulate the blood circulation flow in the chin area. Helping to firm, repeat nightly.

GETTING RID OF CELLULITE

The combination of weight loss, exercise, and massaging will remove cellulite. Just dieting or exercising alone will not rid you of all cellulite. Cellulite is fat deposits in certain areas of the body. The most common areas are the buttocks and the upper, outer thighs. Most of us know what cellulite looks like: it is rippling fat that causes the skin to appear dimpled. Massaging the area that has the cellulite will help loosen and break up the fat. Exercising after the massage is important because exercising increases your blood circulation and helps your body to eliminate the fatty deposits more rapidly.

DO You not Know that your body is a temple of the Holy Ghost, who is in you, whom you have received from God, you are not your own? For you are bought at price therefore honor GOD in your body and in your spirit, which are God's

1 Corinthians 6

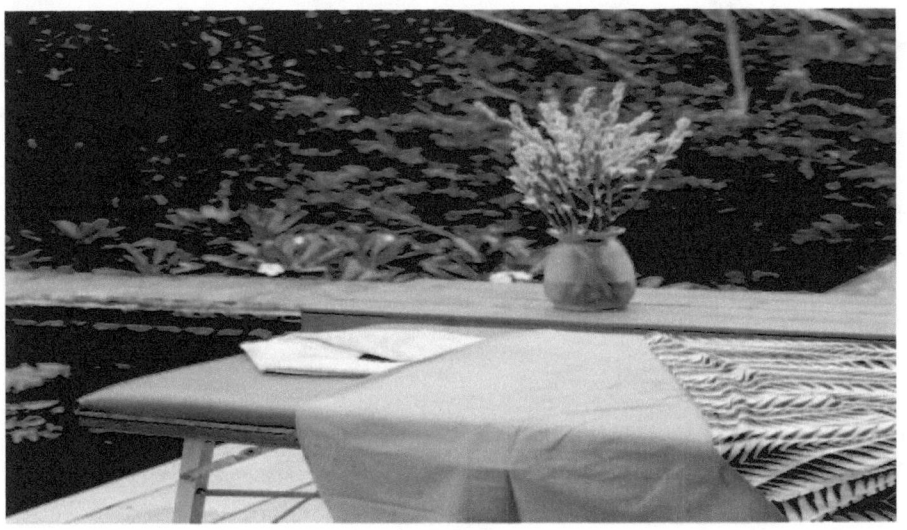

Giving Yourself a Massage

To give yourself a massage, begin first with well-oiled or moistened hands, so that they easily and freely move along your skin. Gently and slowly, start to knead your skin, gradually increasing pressure to influence more blood flow to the desired areas. Massaging always upward and inward towards the heart is important. As you are massaging up the legs and body go inward towards the heart even on the arms. Relax briefly afterwards but do not fall asleep because you will need to follow up with exercises to help tone.

Bath Time Is Healing Time

Baths are well known to calm and relieve stress. Most of us do enjoy a nice hot bath, and most of us are taking on far too much stress even for the best of us. Stress will rob your immune system and upset your physical and emotional state. Since the skin is closely connected to your nervous system it will respond to emotional upsets in various ways. The trick is to keep your peace no matter what. A relaxing bath can do wonders. Be sure the products you use to treat and feed your skin are free of chemicals. Fragrance is very important to relaxing; experiment with your essential oils, and remember a little is all you need... for a little goes a long way.

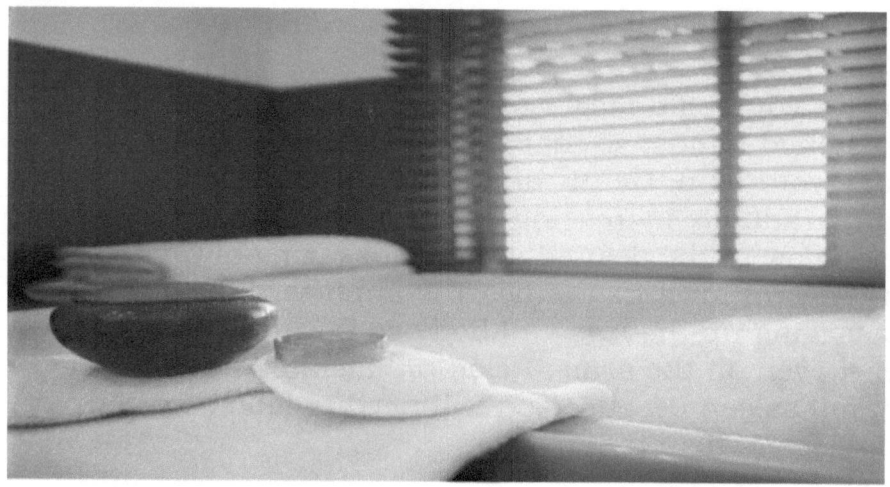

Easy milk bath

One cup of powder milk
¼ cup olive oil
Tablespoon rose oil
Two teaspoons gardenia oil

Place power milk in strainer or stocking
And place under the running tap.
Then add oils to bath water
Enjoy!

Note: after your hot bath or shower, moisturize your skin well as hot water is drying to the skin.

Milk is very nourishing for the skin; it naturally hydrates and restores vitamins and antioxidants.
Organic milk has about twice as much nutrients as regular.

Bubble Milk bath

1/3 cup powder milk
1/4 cup mineral water
1/8 cup coconut
Two tablespoons apricot oil
Two tablespoons jojoba oil
Mix together, keep in glass bottle
Shake before each use, store in refrigerator, will keep a
week or so.

Joy Joy!
Finally you've come and so generously!
filling in this empty shell so completely
I thank you Jesus
 for your love so undeserving
        I thank you father
Of my joy your hope is within me!

Queen Esther herbal bath
(fresh leaves are best)

One tablespoon grape seed oil
One tablespoon Neroli essential
One tablespoon virgin olive oil
One tablespoon myrrh essential oil
One teaspoon rose oil
One teaspoon frankincense
One teaspoon lavender essential oil
One teaspoon vanilla oil
One teaspoon citrus essential oil
¼ cup sage leaves
¼ hyssop leaves
¼ cup Rosemary leaves
¼ cup mint leaves
¼ cup lavender flowers
¼ cup heather flower
¼cup rose petals
2 bay and hyssop leaves
Boiling hot water
After much studying, it was revealed that
Queen Esther most likely bathe in a
Similar treatment like this, Place leaves and petals in
large bowl add water to herbs enough to cover and let
steep about 10 minutes to make a strong tea. Dispose of
leaves and add oils to the tea. Makes two treatments,
prepare a nice batch up and store in glass container until
ready to use.

Queen Esther bath #2

Is a blend penetrating natural oils and Herbs.
Mix your oils together first and stored in glass or ceramic
container until ready to use. 16.0z
one cup soy milk
One tablespoon sweet almond oil
One tablespoon olive oil
One tablespoon carrot seed essential oil
One tablespoon tea tree oil
One teaspoon orange blossom essential oil
One teaspoon lavender essential oil
One teaspoon rose oil
½ teaspoon black currant seed oil
½ teaspoon grape seed oil
½ teaspoon frankincense essential
½ teaspoon myrrh essential oil
¼ teaspoon gardenia extract
A few drops of sage extract
A few drops of comfrey extract
A few drops cucumber extract
A few bay leaves
A couple lemon wedges
A cinnamon stick
Mix all ingredients together place in container until ready
to use. Use as a Moisturizing bath oil treatment or as
daily moisturizer. Studies revealed that Queen Esther
probably, bathe in a similar bath treatment.
It is quite a bit of ingredients but it is worth it for your
wonderful skin. Treat yourself!

Milk and lavender

1/3 cup powder milk
¼ mineral water
¼ cup sunflower oil
Two tablespoons lavender essential oil
1/8 cup primrose oil
One teaspoon jasmine essential oil
Mix all ingredients, stored in glass bottle, shake before use. enjoy!

Oatmeal bath

One cup raw oats
One tablespoon sweet almond oil
One tablespoon jojoba oil
One tablespoon rose hip oil
One teaspoon and a half gardenia oil

Place raw oats in stocking or strainer; immerge it in 3 cups of water for about an hour, prepare bath water. Squeeze water out of the oatmeal dispose of oats, pour oatmeal water into your awaiting bath water, add oils, and enjoy your bath time. This recipe goes way back for many of us it is known as the oat soak., this recipe is one treatment.

— ✳ ~

Balm of Gilead
One cup of natural floral potpourri
¼ cup hyssop leaves
Two tablespoon grape seed oil
One tablespoon St John's-wort oil extract
One teaspoon comfrey extract
¼ teaspoon lemon essential oil

Place potpourri and hyssop in strainer and cover with boiling hot water, steep for one hour, dispose of leaves adding your oils and extract. A cleansing and healing bath enjoy!

Stress relieving dip
 You may use tea bags with this treatment

¼ mineral or Epsom salt
¼ cup chamomile tea leaves
¼ cup mint tea leaves
¼ cup apricot oil
Two teaspoon eucalyptus oil
Place leaves in strainer and place in running bath water, pour in oils. Get in, relax and enjoy your bath

Detox and heal

½ cup mineral sea salt
½ cup pure aloe vera gel or juice
1 ½ tablespoon tea tree oil
1 ½ tablespoon seaweed or bladder wrack extract
One teaspoon rosemary extract
½ teaspoon cypress essential oil

Mix salt and aloe vera together, place in strainer add it along with oils and extract to your bath water, now relax and enjoy your soak. Helps to cleanse heal and soften skin.

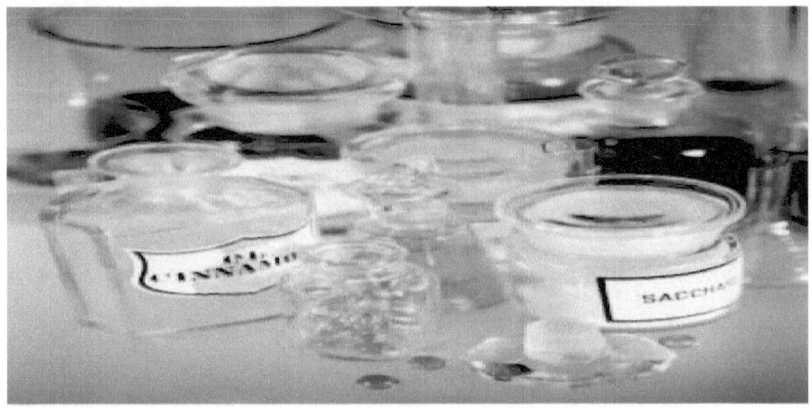

─ ✽ ∼

Jesus you're the one for me

Jesus you're the one for me
Oh, happy day,
he set me free
and Gave me life on Calvary
A love so pure I just believe
Oh Jesus you're the One for me

When no one cared
you came around
and healed my wounds
And holds me now
your righteous path
I'm heaven bound
cause Jesus you're the One for me

The path I take
no looking back
my friends all say what's up with that?
My season changed,
to hope and peace
Oh Jesus you're the one for me.!

─ ✽ ∼

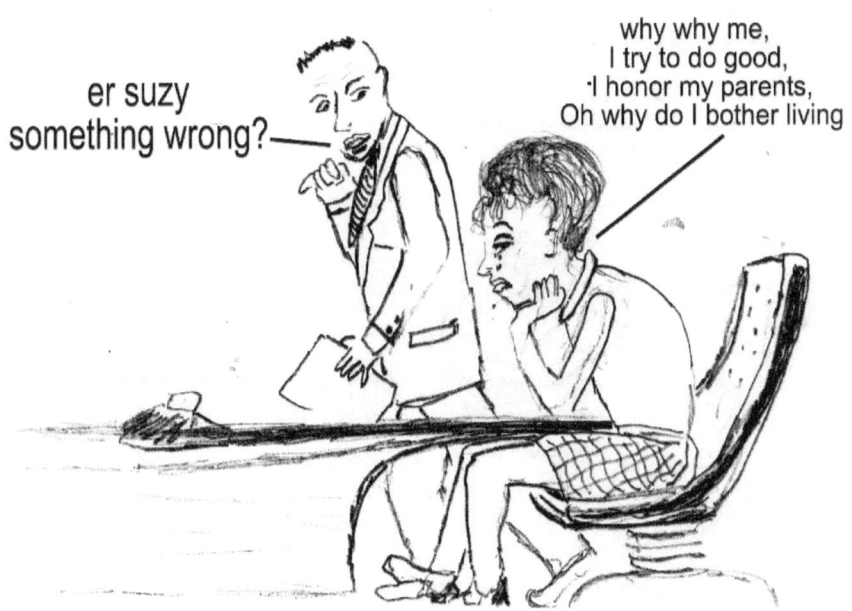

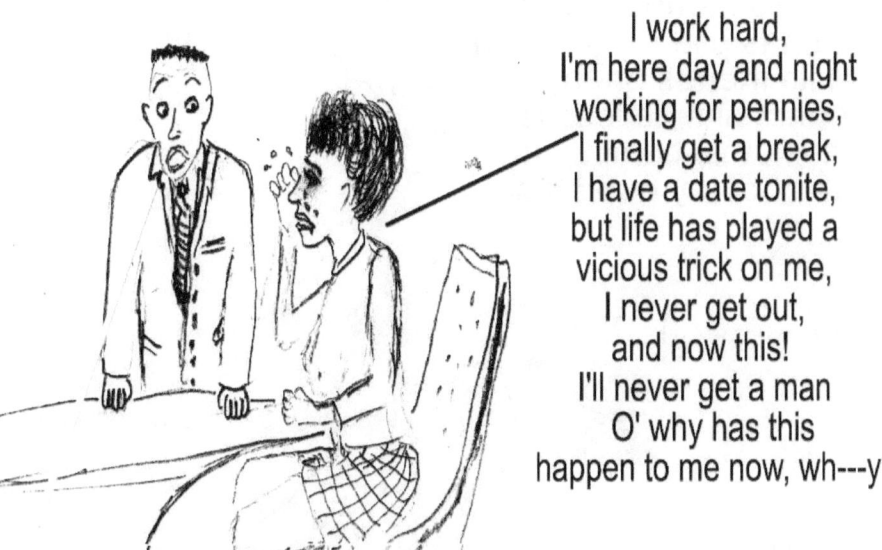

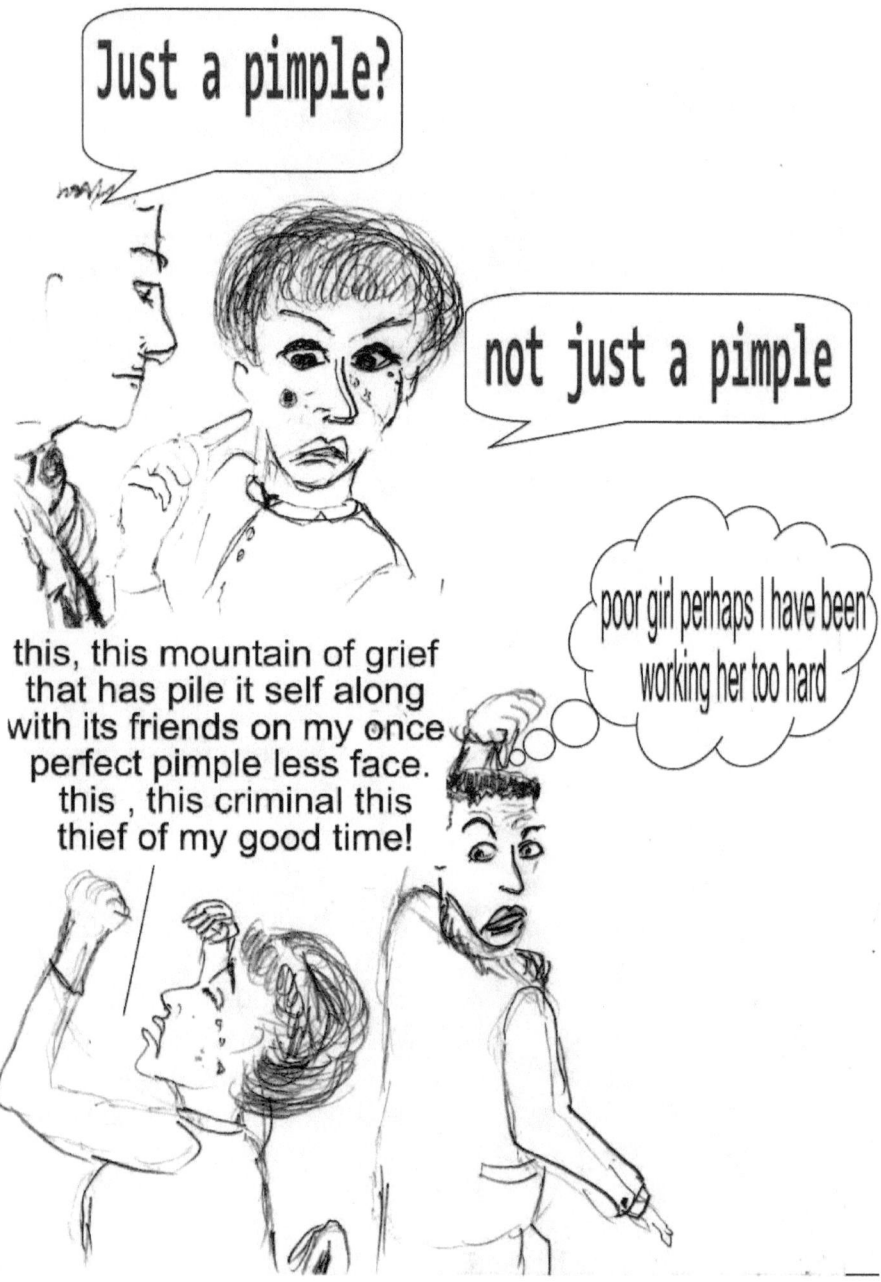

The Vine and the branch

O Lord since you are the vine and I am the
branch, I must stay connected by
more than a glance

Yours words and nourishment must flow in
me where, it's evident that others –
may see, love bursting sprouts blooming
uniquely

O Lord my GOD what more can I say, in you
I have what I need every day, and let the
life you've given to me, be a sweet
smell you savor lovingly

I am the vine ye are the branches: he that
abideth in me and I in him the same
bringeth forth much fruit. For without me
ye can do nothing

John 15

Staying connected

Staying connected is easy you see
just fall in love with Jesus completely

and love is a beautiful thing!
for that is what GOD is and he will
always be

So keep your connection flowing and strong,
you may fall down but it's not
for long

that connection will bring you back to
degree just how good GOD really is to
you and me

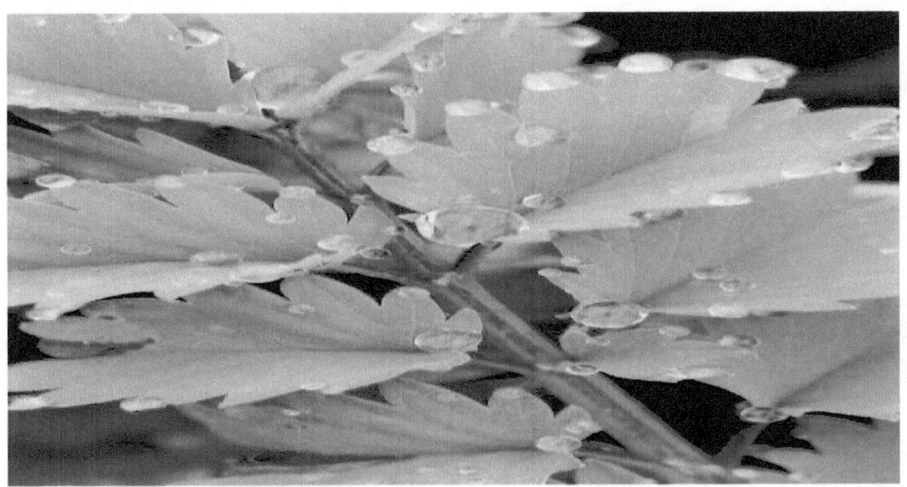

I love the rain or when it snows or when the
sun shines fully glows I'm thankful for your
gift to me, you changed my life abundantly
you given more then I can say and I'm
grateful Father for every day!

Even there your hand shall guide me your
right hand will hold me fast
Psalm 139

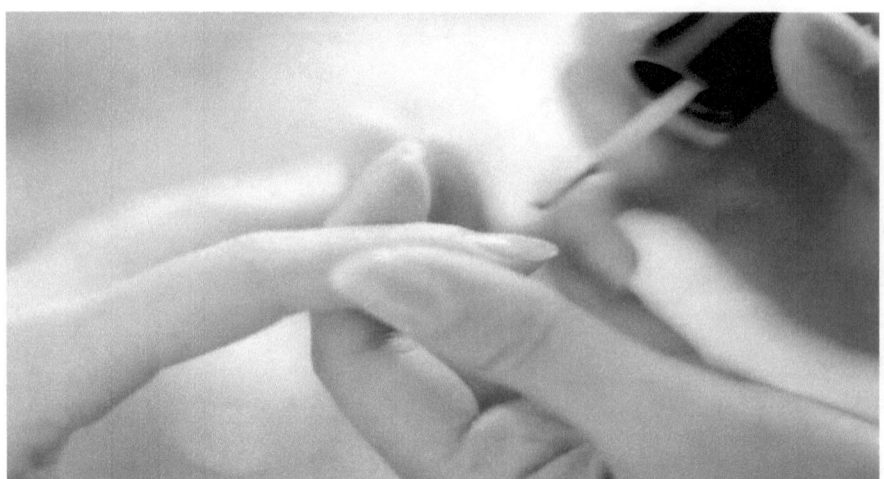

NAILS

Your nails, hair, and skin are made up of a protein substance called keratin. Our nails are made up of different layers. The top layer is called the nail plate. The layer right beneath the nail is called the nail bed, a very soft skin that nourishes the nail plate through blood vessels. Then there is the cuticle, the skin that seals the nail to the skin and also works to keep dirt and other foreign matter from the matrix. The matrix is where the cells for the nail plate are reproduced.

GIVING YOUR SELF A MANICURE

Prepare bowl, for soaking your fingertips.
Fill bowl with warm water and add a squirt of hair
conditioner a teaspoon of fresh lemon juice. Then remove
old nail polish from your nails. Next, follow these
instructions:

1. Soak your fingertips in warm lemon water for 5
minutes
2. Remove and begin to file and shape your nails using
the smooth sides a of the emery board trying not to file
the sides or corners too much.
3. Filing your nails with even strokes in one direction at a
time not back and forth.
4. Apply cuticle cream or oil, massaging in and the entire
hand, pushing your cuticle gently back
5. Clean debris from under or around nails.
6. Gently clip or trim excess skin or enlarged cuticle
7. Rinse hands in warm water, dry
8. Apply nail conditioner and polish
9. Remember to wear gloves while doing your chores to
protect your manicure so it will last longer.

— ✳ —

Homemade hand cream

One tablespoon shea butter
Teaspoon apricot oil
Teaspoon aloe vera gel
½ teaspoon lavender essential oil
½ teaspoon rose hip oil

Blend all together and massage into hands, This one is so easy we will make up a large batch of this and share with all, has healing and anti-aging benefits.

Into your hands I commit my spirit thou hast redeemed me o LORD God of truth. My times are in your hands

Psalm 31

— ✳ —

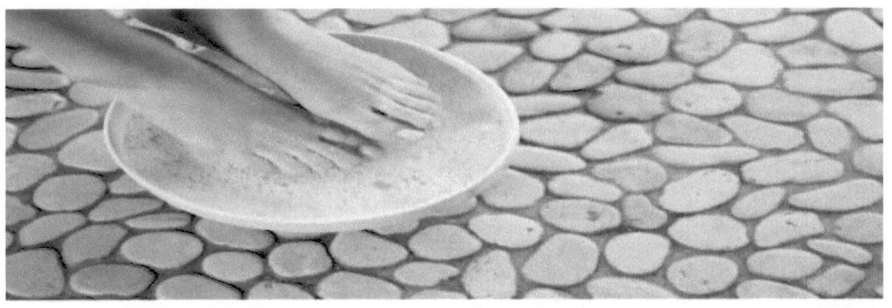

Your word is a lamp to my feet and a light
unto my path
Psalm 119

to give light to them that sit in darkness and
in the shadow of death , to guide our feet
into the way of peace

Luke

135

- ✖ ~

GIVING YOURSELF A PEDICURE

Prepare a tub of warm soapy water to soak your feet. Add about ¼ cup Epsom salt or baking soda and a few drops of a fragrance essential oil and hair conditioner.

1. Remove old polish from nails
2. Soak feet in water
3. Using a callus remover and loofa, scrub away calluses and hardened dead skin from your feet, paying special attention to your heels
4. Exfoliate, rubbing gently on feet with stone, loofa etc..
5. Removing one foot while the other, remains in the warm water. Begin to clean trim and file nails
6. Repeat with the other foot, moisten heel and toes
   w/aloe vera gel
7. Apply nail conditioner and polish
8. Once dry apply petroleum jelly/moisturizer to feet and put on a pair of socks. You can do this last step at night before bed.

How beautiful your sandal feet O prince's daughter
Your graceful legs are like jewels
The work of a craftsman Hands

Song of Solomon

Exfoliate feet

One tablespoon Epsom salt
Tablespoon coconut milk
½ tablespoon lanolin
½ tablespoon extra virgin oil
A few drops of lavender essential oil

Mix all ingredients together rub over entire feet paying special attention to heels.
Rinse and apply moisturizer as usual

Foot cream

One tablespoon warmed vegetable glycerin
A Teaspoon coconut oil
A Teaspoon lanolin
½ teaspoon beeswax
½ teaspoon lavender essential oil

Place all ingredients except lanolin and glycerin in a double boiler or pan on low heat melt wax into oil stir in lanolin and finally vegetable glycerin, let stand to set, use freely to soften feet.

Beautiful hair

The hair is made up of the same substance your nails are
made of, that substance is keratin. Like your nails your
hair is combined of dead skin cells. The hair root itself is
the dermis layer of your skin. There at the hair root are
living cells merging from them are dead skin cells that are
being pushed through the hair follicle to the surface of
the skin, thus giving your hair growth and length. Most
people have about 75,000 to 125,000 hair follicles on
their head each one providing a single strand of hair
through the follicle opening, the pore. The hair is made of
two main layers, the cuticle layer and the cortex layer.
The hair is constantly reproducing itself though; this
process depends on the health, the age, and a person's
heredity background.

But the very hairs of your head are
numbered. So don't be afraid you are
worth more then many sparrows

Matthews 10

THE DIFFERENT STAGES OF HAIR

Under twenty
Because of the increase of oil in the skin during this time the hair is normally a bit oily and may need to be shampoo often. But in general hair should be vibrant and flowing with production on the rise.

Twenty to thirty five
Hair should be thick and radiant and if its damage it can easily be nurse back to health. During pregnancy the female body produces large amounts of estrogen this process will give assistance in the production of hair and nails. After the pregnancy about four to six months afterwards women will notice some hair loss, this is due to the sudden decrease in estrogen. But all in all hair should be vibrant and flowing

Forty+
Some strands may possibly be grey and there may be thinning. And perhaps menopause is approaching if so, a women's natural estrogen declines and her body's androgen (male hormones) appears to want to increase its role. Some women may notice more facial hair, but remember you can revitalize or maintain its health the control knob is in your hand.

GOOD HEALTHY HAIR CARE TIPS

There are so many things that we do to our hair. For instance, coloring chemical perms, blow drying, hot combs and flat irons, curling styling etc. Unfortunately these are all negative actions. It is good to know there are just as many positive things we can do to help the hair regenerate itself... in fact, there are many.

1. Avoid shampoos with harsh detergents. Instead, choose a mild cleanser. Detergents are drying to your scalp and hair.

2. Look for natural products that contain herbs and minerals for example: Indian hemp, rosemary, horsetail, silica, sage, and pantheon. With continuous use your hair will become healthier thicker with shine and more manageability.

3. Remember to drink plenty water your hair needs the water to aid cells in delivering oxygen other nutrients to it.

4. Try not to untangle your wet hair with a brush, as this can damage your hair. Use instead a wide tooth comb, combing through your hair in small sections, ever so gently, to avoid breakage.
5. When choosing a brush, soft, round natural bristles are the best.

6. Avoid over use of blow dryers, heated rollers, flat irons, extensive hair braiding, and tight ponytails, as these actions, when overused, will dry hair and/or irritate the scalp causing hair breakage.

7. Soy bean proteins give your hair life and help in hair repair and growth

8. Drinking Indian hemp and or horse tail in
Tea it is excellent for cell renewal, and aids your hair in thickening and increasing its productions, with continuous use.

9. Exercising increases blood circulation and your hair will love it. Also brushing your hair stimulates hair growth. Another way to increase the blood circulating in your head is to do headstands if you can, full or partial. Simply lay across your bed on your back, letting your shoulders and head hang over the edge. Relax in that position for about 15 minutes a day. This will help oxygenate your hair and will stimulate hair growth.

10. For natural highlights, rinse your hair in fresh lemon juice or hydrogen peroxide.

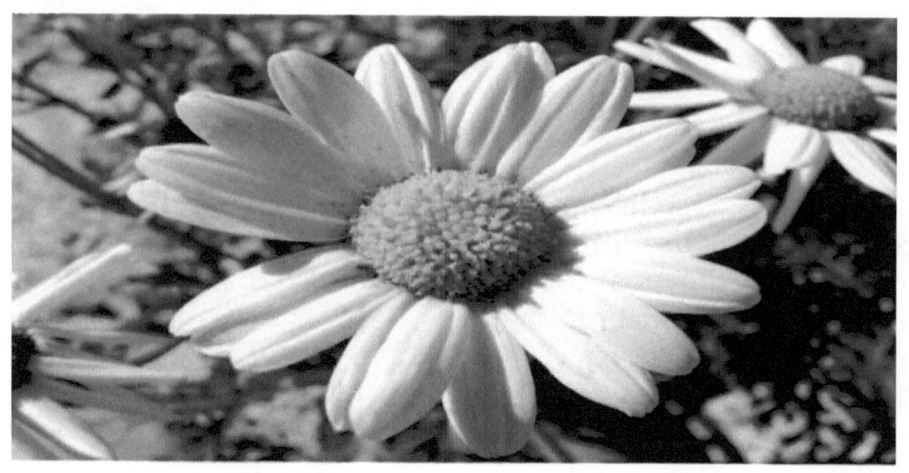

THOU ART FAIR
MY LOVE
THERE IS NO SPOT
IN
THEE

Song Solomon

Woman of Hope

Woman of hope where are you going?

Are your eyes on him? Are you planting?
are you sowing? Are you giving what you got,
reaping the Good land?

Trusting the Lord yielding to his Plan?

The Lord loves you, pay attention he is Calling,
so you better get up and you better Get going,

Woman of hope I saw your eyes today They were
crying I think, Then you went on Your way

Then I saw you smiling too, and I wondered My
darling just who are you?

For you are Purposely driven doing his good,
Talking Good news, helping when you could,

Woman of hope, yes I know who you are
You are me,
A child of the most high GOD

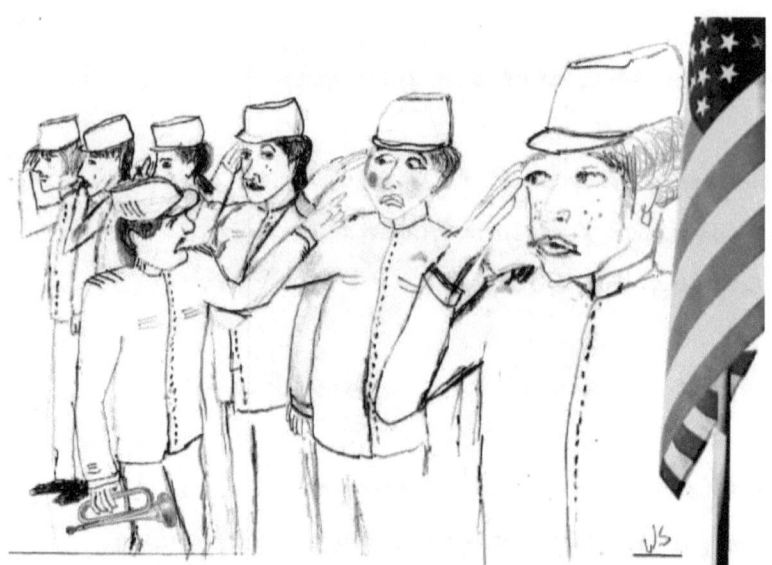

hey private that pimple is standing at attention more then you!

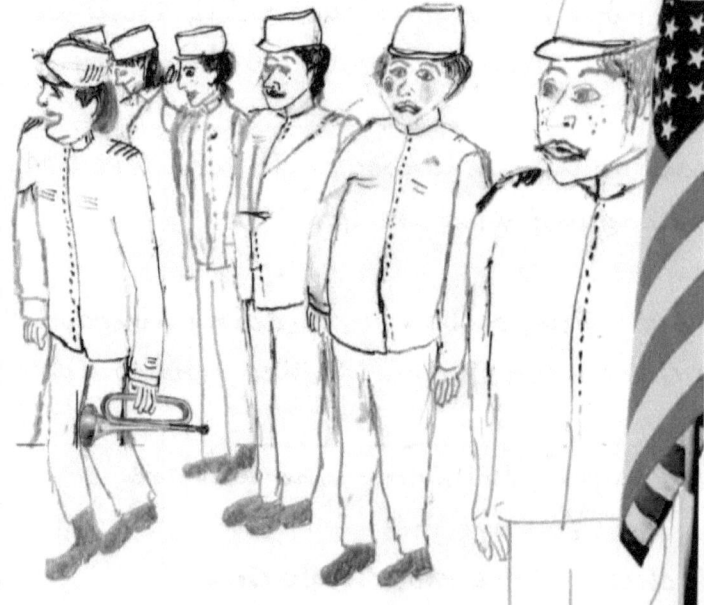

I'm going to give you girlie's something and one day your gonna thank me.

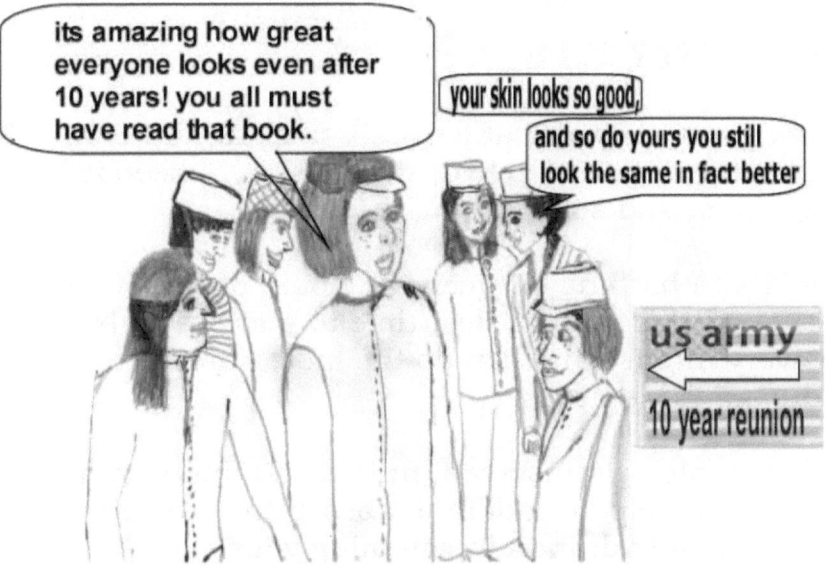

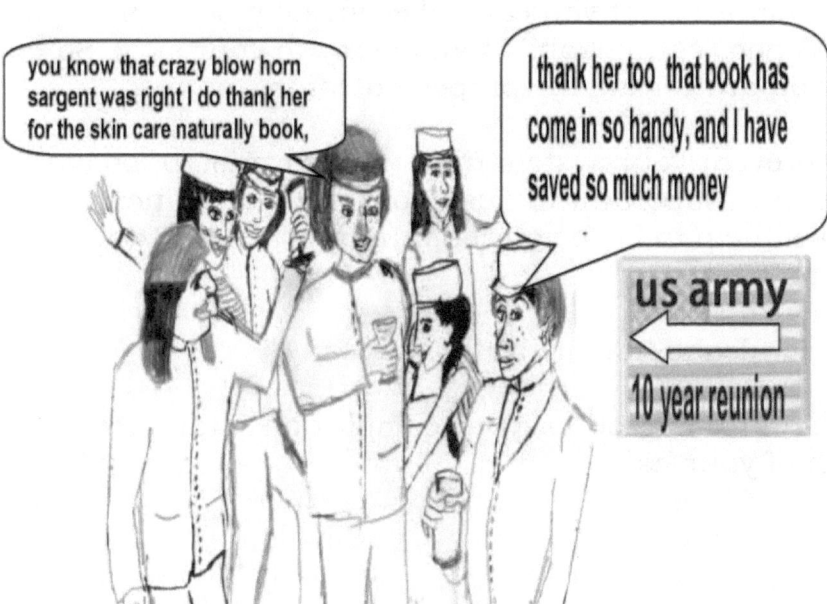

100+ BEAUTY TIPS

1. Drink plenty of water at least six to eight Full 8 0z glasses every day to help hydrate the skin to keep it looking moist and soft

2. Avoid sun bathing between the hours of Eleven and two. Though this may be Best time to sun bathe, but the sun is very intense and can do the most damage to your skin during these hours.

3. Before applying sunscreen, mist with mineral water, the water will help Your skin to absorb the sunscreen and give additional hydration in softening your skin, as the sun is very drying.

4. Remember what you eat will eventually be seen on your skin. A poor eating habit is an enemy to your skin. So be sure you are getting the proper nutrition and rest.

5. To prevent your system from re-absorption of body waste. It is important to flush your system frequently. This will help to keep your skin happy, healthy, and blemish free.

6. Avoid alcohol it dehydrates the skin.

7. Vitamin B is good for your complexion. It improves the health of your hair.

8. Plucking your eyebrows with tweezers can be painless. Try numbing your brow first with ice.

9. For bright strong eyes, try eye exercises.

10. Vaseline or petroleum jelly is an excellent moisturizer and can reduce wrinkles when apply under eye.

11. Home-made lip-gloss, mix a little of your favorite lipstick with petroleum jelly, store in small container.

12. Try baby lotion or coconut oil for gently removing make-up.

13. For fuller moist looking lips massage a good night cream into your lips at night.

14. Natural beer baths will replenish nutrients to your skin.

15. Zinc, the mineral, will promote your collagen restoration in the skin.

16. Eating avocado's helps your skin to produce collagen. Collagen gives your skin a healthy, smooth appearance.

17. Broccoli, alfalfa sprouts, cabbages, and are full of anti-aging properties.

18. Blueberries contain antioxidants properties that reduce wrinkles and helps prevent sagging.

19. Watermelon has vitamin A & C Selenium zinc and Vitamin E, just what your skin needs.

20. Fish, and soybeans, nuts and beans, have anti-aging properties and they help the skin remain healthy and youthful looking.

21. Potassium (bananas) helps remove dark circles from under the eyes. When mashed and applied on the skin under the eyes

22. Fresh slice cucumbers on the eyes will help fade dark circles under the eyes.

23. Fresh raw sliced potato, on the eyes will help fade dark circles.

24. Eating parsley takes away bad breath.

25. For whiter teeth, brush your teeth with apple cider and baking soda

26. For bright white teeth mix and mash a strawberry with baking soda and brush.

27. Mist face with mineral water throughout the day to hydrate and it helps your makeup last a little longer.

28. To condition eyelashes and eyebrows, warm slightly a little virgin olive oil, using a cotton swab dip into the oil and begin to clean your lashes and brows with it. Your lashes will appreciate this treatment will promote hair growth for your lashes and brows.

29. Hot oil treatment for hair, warm two tablespoons of extra virgin olive oil. Massage into hair the cover your head with a shower cap for 15 minutes. Then shampoo as usual.

30. For shining hair add a little baking soda to your shampoo.

31. Conditioner for dry hair: try an avocado mashed and mix with an egg white or mayonnaise. Massage for 10 minutes and rinse out. Restores luster and shine to hair.

32. Conditioner for dry hair, mayonnaise mixed with sweet almond or avocado oil. Massage in hair for 10 minutes, the cover with shower cap for 10 minutes. Shampoo as usual

33. Instant help for hair with split ends. Apply a little night cream to hair ends at night. Or massage jojoba oil into scalp and hair for 10 minutes, then rinse, restores natural nutrients luster and shine, and reduce split ends.

34 Coconut oil is absorb by the skin easily, and it has anti- aging properties

35. To detoxify, your skin boil some fresh rosemary and thyme, let cool a little, dipping loofahs or natural brush in warm tea water firmly yet gently brush your skin all over with even strokes. This will help eliminate toxins by stimulating the lymphatic system and improve blood circulation, because it also helps to remove dead skin cells. Your skin will love it! Shower or bath afterwards

36. To get rid of blemishes or acne mash and mix a few aspirins a little honey and mineral water, make a paste and apply to pimple over night. In the morning pimple should be gone or at least much better.

37. Dab tea tree oil on pimples to help fight kill the bacteria and helps heal the inflammation.

38. To fight acne, mix and mash an apple and one tablespoon raw honey. Apply to face or pimples leave on 5-10 minutes. Rinse clean

39. Peel and sliced garlic, and rub slices of garlic on pimples. The garlic helps fight the eruptions.

40. Exercising increases blood circulation oxygen intake and improves the skin health. Also exercising reduces cellulite, firms and promotes a more youthful appearance.

41. Sweating when exercising, is the process of your body cooling its self. Your skin contains two types of glands one produces oil the other secretes sweat. Sweating helps eliminate bacteria from the body. 1/3 of body toxins are eliminated through sweating.

42. A stimulating firming toner
    One tablespoon ginseng root extract
    One tablespoon aloe vera gel
    Eight ounces of mineral water
    Put all ingredients in spritz bottle, shake & mist.

43. Anti-aging refreshing mist
    One tablespoon ginseng root extract
    One tablespoon glycerin
    One tablespoon mint oil
    1 1/2 teaspoon fresh lemon juice
16 0z of mineral water, mix all in spray bottle and mist skin frequently with this anti-aging serum. Carry this mist with you and mist skin often, will restore moisture and antioxidants to skin.

44. Anti-aging body mist
Brew tea w/fresh rosemary and thyme leaves, let cool add equal part carbonated mineral water and a drop of lemon balm essential oil, use a mist bottle, mist body anytime, store in refrigerator. Helps body to detox.

45. Anti-aging for eyes, watermelon slices place over the eyes, help reduce wrinkles, and helps to tone the eye area.

46. Massaging vitamin E oil under and around eye area reduces and prevents wrinkles & crowfeet, softens and smooth's.

47. Rinsing your skin with mineral water nourishes and softens it.

48. For lightly fragrance skin
In mist bottle, filled with carbonated mineral water add a few drops of essential oil, lavender or myrrh, mist skin anytime oils also tones the skin.

49. For lightly fragrance sensitive skin. In mist bottle, filled with carbonated mineral water add a few drops of rose essential oil, rose oil is very effective, excellent for dry aging or sensitive skin. And the fragrance is desirable.

50. Healing body mist, add together eight ounces of carbonated mineral water, one tbsp pure aloe gel, a few drop of rose hips oil, shake before using. Mist skin anytime has healing and anti-aging properties, promotes healthy skin.

51. To lighten hair or for highlights, rinse hair in fresh lemon juice.

51. Beer conditioner, rinse hair in natural beer, helps restore health and shine to hair.

52. After shampooing, use protein base conditioner to help restore natural oils.

53. For a few gray strands of hair cover with mascara.

54. To help repair dry brittle hair, rinse in cool brew chamomile tea.

— ❈ ~

55. Yogurt hair conditioner, apply plain yogurt to clean wet hair leave on five minutes, rinse. Helps to strengthen hair and restore a natural balance.

56. for soft smooth skin around the eyes. Gently massage a little mayonnaise under eyes nightly, reduces wrinkles.

57. For soft smooth skin around the eyes gently massage Castor oil under the eyes nightly. Reduces wrinkles

58. For smooth skin around the eyes massage almond oil gently daily.

59. Dark green vegetables help to give you bright healthy eyes.

60. for soft smooth skin around the eyes mixed petroleum jelly and vitamin E oil, apply to skin nightly reduces wrinkles and sagging.

61. For bright eyes, place cool, wet used tea bags, over eyes, helps reduce puffiness and darkens eyelashes.

62. Remove make up gently, with sesame oil

63. For soft youthful skin massage coconut oil into skin nightly.

64. For removing or fading age or dark spots, rub a lemon wedge over skin every other day.

65. To lighten knees and elbows before bed, apply fresh lemon juice to them.

66. Exfoliate the feet, mix shea butter with kosher salt or sugar; you can add mint oil to make it fun massage into feet & rinse.

67. Skin conditioner make a soft paste with power milk and coconut oil, rub into skin try to work up lather, rinse in shower

68. Body scrub, mix finely ground kosher salt with extra virgin olive oil and a little fresh orange juice and orange peels. Rub over entire body avoid genital area, rinse in shower. Reveals soft new skin

69. Body scrub, mix plain yogurt and wheat germ, vanilla oil, massage in, rinse in shower. Reveals soft new skin

70. Body scrub, mix finely ground kosher salt with aloe vera gel, jojoba oil and a few drop of mint oil, rub into skin gently, rinse in shower.

71. For extra soft skin, before bed massage petroleum jelly into skin and put on cotton pajamas and socks.

72. For soft youthful face and hands massage sweet almond oil or extra virgin olive oil, into your face and hands nightly.

73. For soft feet before bed rub petroleum jelly into feet pay special attention to calluses, sleep with socks on

74. For help with oily hair try shampoos with herbs, fruit juice or extracts.

75 Test a small amount first, before using and ingredient on skin.

76. Fighting pimples, apply peroxide on pimple till cleared.

77. Dab apple cider on pimple till it clears up

78. Mix baking soda and mineral water make a paste, apply to pimple.

79. Witch hazel on pimple will help to heal from the eruption.

80. Dab lime juice on pimple, to help get rid of it.

81. For soft hands mix kosher salt almond oil, and a few drops of lavender essential oil.

83. Acne mask, make a paste mixing wheat flour or corn starch with lime juice and tea tree oil, apply to skin, let dry, rinse.

84. Apple's are a natural cleanser for healthy teeth. Apple's help to remove plague, rinse mouth after eating.

85. Celery is a natural cleanser for teeth it helps remove plague.

86. Eating strawberries cleans teeth, rinse mouth afterwards.

87. Rinsing mouth frequently will help cut down on bacteria and bad breath.

88. Green tea may help you lose weight.

89. Tea & coffee may stain teeth.

90. For healthy teeth, vitamin A, D & C is necessary and the mineral calcium

91. Foods high in vitamin A, dark green vegetables, yellow fruits, fish& eggs.

92. Foods high in cancer fighting vitamin D are fish, egg yolks omega 3.

93. Foods high in C vitamin are citrus fruits and melons.

94. The mineral Calcium is found in dairy products, broccoli, tofu, beans and nuts

95. For bright healthy eyes eat garlic, avocado asparagus, beans, onions and of course carrots.

96. For healthy nails be sure to eat garlic, eggs, fish flax seed oil, nuts & spinach

97. For shiny healthy hair be sure to include in your diet, fish dark vegetables iron zinc, beans and biotin.

98. Eating your spinach and massaging spinach juice, mix with aloe vera gel and vitamin E oil; massage nightly on spider veins, will help rid you of them

99. Smoking depletes skin of its natural oils, skin will eventually appear lifeless.

100. After washing face always splash with cold water, the cold water will help close pores and tone skin.

   Soy milk can be substituted for the **goat**
101. **Ancient Egyptian beauty wash #1**
      Two tablespoons goat milk
      One drop myrrh essential oil
      One drop gardenia oil mix, wash and rinse.

102. Ancient beauty wash #2
     Tablespoon fresh goat milk
     ½ teaspoon fresh lemon or lime juice
     A drop or two of rose oil mix, wash and rinse.

103. Ancient beauty wash #3
     Two tablespoon fresh cream
     ½ teaspoon fresh orange juice
     A drop of frankincense essential oil mix,
     wash and rinse.

104. Ancient beauty scrub #1
     Two tablespoons buttermilk
     One tablespoon ground wheat germ
     One teaspoon fresh ground rosemary leaves
     A drop of frankincense essential oil
     mix, wash and rinse.

105. Ancient beauty scrub #2
     Two tablespoons goat milk
     One tablespoon raw oats
     One teaspoon virgin olive oil
     A drop of myrrh essential oil
     A drop of frankincense oil
     mix, wash and rinse.

106. Ancient beauty scrub #3
> Fresh dairy Cream
> Fresh ground rosemary
> Fresh ground bay leaves
> Fresh ground thyme
> A few drops of rose essential oil
> Use your best judgment regarding portions,
> mix, wash and rinse

107. Ancient body scrub
> Butter or animal fat
> Raw sugar
> Vanilla scented oil
> Fresh ground thyme
> Again use your best judgment regarding
> portions, apply over body rinse in shower,
> Leaves skin feeling soft and moisten.

108. Ancient bath treatment
> One quart goat milk
> ¼ cup virgin olive oil
> A few drop of lavender essential oil
> Fresh rosemary leaves
> Add all items to running bath water,
> moisturizes and restores nutrients to skin.

109. Ancient bath treatment #2
        ½ cup grape seed oil
        ¼ cup jojoba oil
        One teaspoon citrus essential oil
        Fresh oregano leaves
        Fresh rosemary leaves

Place leaves in strainer under running tap place other ingredients in bath water and enjoy. This is a moisturizing, bath with anti- aging benefits.

110. When leaving bath or shower use damp wash cloth or sponge to pat dry your skin, then apply your moisturizer to your damp skin. That will help to keep your skin soft and supple.

111. Remember this rule, if you can't pronounce it you shouldn't eat it and if you can't eat it, you shouldn't put it on your skin.

112. For flawless skin, try detox-ing your body and clean your colon, drink lots of water and take a fast from artificial sweeteners and Ingredients, including caffeine and nicotine. Begin to eat fresh natural foods.

113. During a fast, before bathing,
take a natural brush dab in oregano oil or sage oil,
brush your skin ever so gently to help pull impurities out,
this will tone and reduce cellulite if any, then shower as usual.

Hawaii beauty secrets

114. Use coconut oil to remove makeup, coconut oil easily removes makeup and restores vital nutrients to your dewy skin.

115. Coconut pineapple wash

¼ cup fresh pineapple juice
¼ cup mineral water
¼ cup coconut oil
¼ cup aloe vera gel

Mix together use twice day. Has anti-aging properties for skin renewal.

116. Simply Coconut wash
½ teaspoon fresh lemon juice
½ teaspoon coconut oil
aloe vera gel can be added
Apply to damp face, work up lather rinse, apply toner.

117. Use banana's to strengthen hair, mash a banana with ¼ cup coconut oil
after shampooing hair, apply banana mix as a conditioner 10 minutes, then rinse.

118. Banana scrub,
One large mashed banana
¼ cup finely ground sea salt
¼ coconut oil

Mash banana till creamy add other ingredients, exfoliate and hydrates skin.

119. Pineapple & papaya mask
¼ cup puree pineapple & papaya together
2 tablespoon wheat flour or red clay
1 tablespoon diary cream
1 teaspoon macadamia oil

Mix, apply rinse after 10 minutes, leaves skin soft and renewed.

120. Papaya cleanser
¼ cup papaya juice
¼ cup mineral water
1 teaspoon E oil
1 teaspoon jojoba oil

Store in refrigerator, a excellent facial cleanse, restores nutrients the enzymes in the papaya will help to remove dead skin cells revealing soft glowing skin.

121. Coconut oatmeal cleanser
½ cup raw oats soaked in one cup of mineral water for a day, remove oats squeezing the water from them. Dispose of oats, and add to oatmeal water,
>   ¼ cup coconut oil
>   ¼ cup aloe vera gel
>   A teaspoon fruit extract
Mix a hydrating cleanser restoring nourishing nutrients.

122. Ginger coconut mask
1 tablespoons puree fresh ginger
1 tablespoon clay or wheat flour
1 ½ tablespoon macadamia oil
A teaspoon papaya juice, warm slightly and apply, let dry then rinse. Gives face a lift leaves skin soft and supple.

123. Mango scrub.
½ well mashed mango
A Tablespoon Finely ground sea salt
A tablespoon vegetable glycerin
A tablespoon coconut oil
One teaspoon rose hip oil

Mix, apply cleans and soften skin.

Lily water: one cup fresh orchids lilies or rose flower petals, place in glass jar with carbonated mineral water just enough to cover it, seal it and store about a week shaking often, drain flower petals off when ready to use water.

124. Lily Fresh- face cleaner
½ cup lily water
Tablespoon aloe vera gel
Tablespoon vegetable glycerin
Two teaspoons sweet almond oil
 ½ teaspoon primrose oil
¼ to ½ teaspoon citrus extract
Store in glass bottle shake before using,
normal skin. A wonderful cleanser!

125. Lily cream- face cleaner
½ cup lily water
½ cup fresh dairy cream
½ teaspoon jojoba oil or coconut
½ teaspoon cucumber seed oil
½ teaspoon fruit extract
½ teaspoon primrose oil
Mix, stored in glass container, hydrates and
softens skin, a moisturizing wash.

Forever Faithful Father

Faithful Lord you are, Faithful Lord my most high
GOD, Your presence is so sweet to me
I thank you my joy my victorious King

I recall the story of Abraham, How he offer Isaac
and a sacrifice lamb He believed you for impossible
things If you did it for him you'll do it for me

So I dance before the father of lights, Oh I dance
before him with all my might
My prayers are answered and all I can say is I love
you Jesus in every way

My Lord you are so faithful to me, You are my life
my world I bless you King, And lift you high for all
to see That forever faithful father you are to me!

Finally beauty comes from the inside, as we have all heard and it's true. Your attitude is an essential matter to beauty. Also what you are thinking will eventually come out of your mouth, to form and direct you.

> Think words that have life and try to keep a good attitude and freely give to others this is true beauty. Choose to think positive even when the odds are against you discard, thoughts that are negative, give no life to them. Remember you are loved and you are wonderfully and uniquely made accept his love today!

We thank you for purchasing this book. We are constantly looking for ways to fund our efforts in assisting the needy. Please know that your purchase is helping thousands of hurting people. Thank you so much for your support!

M.A.W
Missionaries at work

Notes:

www.ingramcontent.com/pod-product-compliance
Lightning Source LLC
Chambersburg PA
CBHW020431290526
45785CB00002B/794